"What's Wrong?" He Asked,

concerned that she had come at this late hour.

"Us," she said.

"Us?" he echoed, stunned. "Heather, there is no 'us.' I'm your foreman; I work for you. You need me to keep this ranch alive, to bring it back up to its former level. You can't sacrifice that. You can't!"

"Must we sacrifice something more important?" Heather asked in a whisper.

To Reid's ears the whisper was a roar.

MONICA BARRIE
is a native of New York State. She has traveled extensively around the world but has returned to settle in New York. A prolific romance writer, Monica's tightly woven emotional stories are drawn from her inherent understanding of relationships between men and women.

Dear Reader:

Silhouette has always tried to give you exactly what you want. When you asked for increased realism, deeper characterization and greater length, we brought you Silhouette Special Editions. When you asked for increased sensuality, we brought you Silhouette Desire. Now you ask for books with the length and depth of Special Editions, the sensuality of Desire, but with something else besides, something that no one else offers. Now we bring you SILHOUETTE INTIMATE MOMENTS, true romance novels, longer than the usual, with all the depth that length requires. More sensuous than the usual, with characters whose maturity matches that sensuality. Books with the ingredient no one else has tapped: excitement.

There is an electricity between two people in love that makes everything they do magic, larger than life—and this is what we bring you in SILHOUETTE INTIMATE MOMENTS. Look for them this May, wherever you buy books.

These books are for the woman who wants more than she has ever had before. These books are for you. As always, we look forward to your comments and suggestions. You can write to me at the address below:

Karen Solem
Editor-in-Chief
Silhouette Books
P.O. Box 769
New York, N.Y. 10019

MONICA BARRIE
Cry Mercy, Cry Love

Silhouette Special Edition
Published by Silhouette Books New York
America's Publisher of Contemporary Romance

SILHOUETTE BOOKS, a Simon & Schuster Division of
GULF & WESTERN CORPORATION
1230 Avenue of the Americas, New York, N.Y. 10020

ISBN: 0-671-53594-3

First Silhouette Books printing May, 1983

10 9 8 7 6 5 4 3 2 1

Map by Ray Lundgren

America's Publisher of Contemporary Romance

Printed in the U.S.A.

To Julia,
Who turns dreams into realities

Cry Mercy,
Cry Love

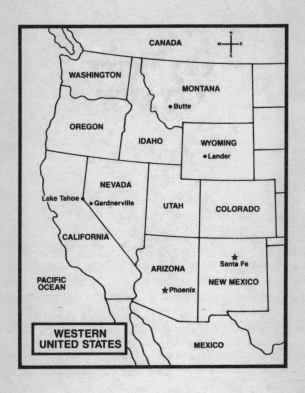

Chapter One

The clay felt soft and pliable in her fingers as Heather Strand began to work it. The clean, earthy scent of the clay filled her senses completely, almost overpowering the other scents around her. The smells of horses, hay, feed, and sweat, mixed with those of the dewy morning, left her, replaced by the smell of the moist clay.

"Ready, Gregg?" Heather asked. A boy of eight stood next to her. His straight wheat-colored hair fell across his forehead, and his small mouth was set in a half-smile. Enormous eyes watched her hands as they worked the clay.

"Yes'm," Gregg replied.

"Have a seat," Heather said as she placed the reddish clay on her work pedestal and began to round it into a rough shape. Gregg watched her work as he moved to the stool and once again looked his father's boss over.

In his eyes Heather Strand seemed more like one of his friends. Gregg was tall for eight, almost five feet. Heather stood only four inches taller. She was dressed like him too—washed-out jeans, boots, and a checked flannel shirt. Her light brown hair was under a straw hat, but Gregg could see the long hair that spilled from beneath it, falling softly past her shoulders.

"Are you comfortable?" Heather asked.

"Yes'm," he replied.

"Gregg, I swear you're starting to sound just like your father."

"Yes'm," Gregg said again, but this time he smiled. He hoped he sounded like his father; he wanted to be like him when he grew up. Gregg's father, Tom Farley, was the best horse breaker on the ranch, and Gregg wanted to be the best breaker in the world.

"Polaris?" Heather called. A low bark was her response as the German shepherd came up to her and rubbed along her leg. "Good boy," she said as she wiped her left hand and scratched the dog behind its ear. "Call him, Gregg. He'll keep you company while I work."

The boy called the dog and Polaris obediently went over to sit next to him. Polaris put his head on Gregg's lap, moving his dark brown eyes upward until he stared directly into the eight-year-old's face. Smiling, Gregg began to stroke the dog's head.

"Miss Heather?"

"Yes, Gregg?"

"Pa says that you're the best sclup . . . I mean, sculterer . . ."

"Sculptor."

"The best . . . sculptor in the world," he finished.

"Why, thank you, Gregg. I do wish I were, but I'm not. What I am trying to do is what I love best."

"Yes'm."

"Gregg, you can move around as much as you want, but just hold still when I tell you to, okay?"

"Okay," he said with a smile as he looked into Heather Strand's soft blue eyes. This was the first time Gregg Farley was going to be Heather's model. Do a "sittin'," his father had told him. He was both excited and puzzled. He was not really sure how she could do what she did, but he also knew that what she did was beautiful. As that thought ran through the young boy's mind, his eyes fell on the sculpture of Polaris, the German shepherd. It was on the other side of the studio, and even as he petted the living dog, he thought he saw the statue smile. Gregg had never seen a sculpture that looked so lifelike.

Then he watched as Heather came over to him and smiled at him. Gregg smiled back as he felt her fingers begin to trace along his face.

Reid Hunter pulled the Land-Rover off the road and stepped down from the front seat. The sun beat down and Reid felt the early spring warmth fill him. His eyes wandered around as he took in the countryside. The tall interlocking mountains displayed their deep emerald green slopes. The land was a mixture of grass and earth that seemed to bid him welcome. Finally his eyes settled on the fence that stretched for miles on the level valley floor. Reid had a good feeling as he climbed back in his vehicle, a better feeling than he'd had in years. This was good land, peaceful and bountiful, and held no memories.

"All right, Miss Strand, you're about to meet your new foreman," he said to himself as his eyes roamed over the mountains again.

Reid knew he would be the first to be interviewed for

the job. He'd known it when he'd picked up the Sunday paper last week and had seen the ad. It had drawn his attention as nothing else had in weeks. The advertisement had been short, to the point, and just what he was looking for.

> FOREMAN/G.M. Wanted for 25,000-acre
> Nevada ranch. Must handle every
> phase of ranch. Send resume and
> references TIMES-BOX 721836R

Reid smiled to himself at the memory. When he'd seen the ad, he'd responded quickly. Two days later, he'd taken a chance, knowing that, no matter what, he wanted that job, or one like it. G.M. positions on small ranches were not that available.

The Tuesday after he'd read the ad he'd called the newspaper. It had been a good ploy and it had worked. He'd gotten the classified operator to divulge the name and address of the advertiser, and he knew he would have the first interview. Again Reid thought of his ploy and of its success.

"*Phoenix Times,* Classified," the operator had said.

"I was wondering if you could help me," Reid had begun, letting authority fill his voice as he spoke. "I placed an ad that ran Sunday. Could you tell me if there's been any response."

"Box number and category?"

"Seven-two-one-eight-three-six-R, Help Wanted."

The operator had put him on hold and three minutes later came back. "There have been five responses, Mr. Strand, and we will be sending these to you on Thursday."

"Wonderful," Reid had replied enthusiastically. "Oh, I just thought of something. Did I give you the ranch address or the postal box delivery?"

"Strand Ranch, Box Two Thirteen, Gardnerville, Nevada."

"Right. Thank you," Reid had replied as he hung up the phone. From there it had taken only three things to accomplish the rest of his plan. The first was the drive to Gardnerville, which was just a few miles outside of Lake Tahoe; the second was to locate the ranch; the third was to call the Strand Ranch and make an appointment.

Today he had the appointment. Reid started up the Land Rover and listened to its powerful engine break the silence of the morning. Ten minutes later Reid drove through the front gate of the Strand Ranch and pulled to a stop in front of the main house. As he reached the ground, a tall, gangly cowboy dressed in work clothes strolled over to him.

"Help you?" he asked.

"I've got an appointment with Miss Strand," Reid informed him. "Reid Hunter," he said as he extended his hand.

The cowboy looked him over critically for a long moment before he took the hand. When he did, Reid felt power within it.

"Tom Farley," he said as he nodded. "Miss Heather's in her studio, workin'."

"Working?" Reid asked with an uplifted eyebrow.

"Go around the main house—you'll see the studio behind it."

"Thank you," Reid said as he started toward the house.

"Hunter," Tom Farley called. Reid stopped and

turned to face the cowboy. "You the same Hunter that worked the Pegasus, in Wyoming?"

"Same one," Reid acknowledged.

"Heard 'bout you. Good luck," Farley said as he turned away and started walking to the corral.

"Did you now?" Reid said to himself as he continued.

When he reached the back of the main house he stopped. A small, partially hidden building stood about fifty feet behind it, looking more like an adobe Indian shack than part of the ranch. The walk itself made Reid pause. It was a five-foot-wide fieldstone pathway, but what made him pause was what lined it. A sculpture was positioned every few feet. Small likenesses of various types of trees and birds stood on pedestals, intermixed with two dogs and other small animals. Reid surveyed each one critically and acknowledged that if they had the color of their living models he would not have been able to tell that they were sculptures.

Near the adobe building were two more sculptures, which were not like the others, but rather more abstract. Reid gazed at them, confused at first, until he let his mind free and stopped trying to put a tag on them. They almost defied description, with curving lines that blended into strong angles. Reid didn't know what they were, but he did know that whoever had made them had created something both breathtaking and beautiful.

Finally Reid reached the building and paused. The door was open and Reid stepped into its frame. His eyes adjusted quickly to the low light and he searched within. His eyes stopped on two figures.

Reid watched silently as the woman worked with the clay. A young boy sat on a stool, his face turned to watch the woman whose fingers molded the clay, as one of his hands absently stroked a large dog. Reid saw the back of Heather Strand. She was not tall, perhaps five four. She had a slender frame, but Reid was not unappreciative of the way her hips flared in the snug-fitting jeans. The straw cowboy hat hid her hair, but what fell to her back caught the light and reflected softly back at him.

As Reid stepped inside, the dog lifted its head and emitted a low growl.

"Don't be shy. If you want to come in, come ahead," Heather instructed. She was used to the people at the ranch coming by when she worked. It seemed to fascinate them, watching her work, and Heather enjoyed the company. If they wanted to talk, she would talk with them. If they just wanted to watch, that was fine with her too. Her art was almost her whole life, and because it was, she was willing to share it with everyone.

But Polaris's next low growl warned her that this visitor was different. The dog knew everyone, and only with a stranger would he growl this way.

"Hush," Heather ordered. Her fingers were molding the ridge of Gregg's chin and she could almost feel the clay as if it were the boy's real skin. As she worked, she spoke to the visitor. "Can I help you?"

"Yes, ma'am, I'm Reid Hunter. I've an appointment with you today."

"Mr. Hunter," Heather said as she dipped her hands into a basin of water and then began to dry them. "Come in," she said. But to Gregg or anyone else who might have heard her her voice seemed different. Heather spent more time drying her hands than was necessary as she tried to concentrate. Reid Hunter's voice had struck something within her. The deep timbre of his voice—the strength in it—resonated within the chambers of her mind and she felt shaken. Heather took a deep breath and turned.

Reid walked toward Heather Strand as she dried her hands. When she turned, he was only two feet away. Reid saw her hand held out and automatically took it within his own. As his fingers closed on it, he looked into Heather's face and his breath caught. Her eyes were the softest blue he had ever seen, and her face was itself a work of art. Her cheekbones were high and Reid knew there was Indian in her blood. Her lips were soft peach and her teeth were an even white that just peaked between her lips. Heather Strand's skin was tanned dark, and Reid could see the laugh lines that creased the corners of her eyes. Reid knew that Heather Strand was a rancher, and one of the most beautiful he'd ever met.

"A pleasure, Mr. Hunter," Heather said as she let go of his hand, giving a silent thanks that her voice had held out. Then, pushing away the strength of her reaction to his voice and the feel of power that had been in his hand, she smiled.

"I hope I'm not interrupting you," Reid said as he looked at the clay that she'd been working on. He could already see a likeness of the young boy on it, and he now knew who had created the beauty that lined the pathway to the studio.

"Of course you are," Heather said with a laugh. "Anything that stops me from working is an interruption, but I do have a ranch that comes first." Heather's smile was infectious, and Reid smiled with her. He watched her eyes as they darted randomly around, never really stopping, and never holding his own gaze after her initial greeting. Then she turned toward the boy and dog. "That's it for today, Gregg. We'll try again during the week, okay?"

"Yes'm," replied the boy as he stood and gave Polaris one final pat. With a smile to Reid, he ran from the studio.

"Boy's in a fearful hurry," Reid commented.

"Wants to watch his father break the pony he's getting next week for his birthday."

"I'd be running too," Reid agreed.

"I didn't expect you so early. Most people don't get to moving around here until afternoon. Saturday night's a big one for the local cowboys," Heather said.

"Yes, ma'am. I came early to get a look around, see what you have here."

"Do you approve?" Heather asked as she went back to the pedestal and took a wet cloth from the basin and covered the form of Gregg's bust.

"It's a nice spread."

"Mr. Hunter, this ranch has been owned by my family for seventy-eight years. We've always run it well and we've always turned a profit. I'm the last of the Strands, unless I have children, and I intend to keep up the standards that have always been a part of this ranch."

Reid was good at understanding what people were saying without listening to their actual words. Heather Strand was saying something, but the way she said it told Reid she meant something else. And Reid felt that what she was saying was more of a challenge than a statement.

Ranching was hard and for a woman even harder. Few women were able to cope with the enormous demands of running a ranch, and those who could were usually harder than the men who worked for them. Heather Strand did not seem to fit into that mold. Reid heard the determination in her voice and saw it echoed on her face as she turned back to face him.

"I can understand your feelings, Miss Strand."

"I don't think so. . . . But if you do come to work here, you will. Shall we go to the house and have some coffee while we talk?"

"After you," Reid responded.

"Polaris!" Heather called. The shepherd came from the stool and went to Heather. A quick scratch under his ear was his reward as Heather began to walk.

Reid watched Heather walk with smooth, confident steps, but he also saw that the dog kept his side pressed against her right leg. As they came out into the daylight, Reid came alongside Heather. Squinting his eyes against the harshness of the sun, Reid looked into Heather Strand's face. Her eyes were still fully open, unsquinting against the powerful noonday sun. With a sudden shock Reid understood why her voice had sounded challenging.

"It must be difficult," he said, ineffectually trying to hide the sadness he felt.

Heather stopped as if struck. She turned sideways to face him and her mouth turned into a hard line. "You're about to lose the job before you get it," she told him.

"No, ma'am. You need me more than I realized."

"I need no one who pities me."

"I don't know you well enough to pity you," Reid informed her in a stiffly formal voice.

"Good. Shall we continue?"

"Yes, ma'am."

"You may call me Heather. Everyone on the ranch does."

"Ask away, Miss Heather," Reid said to her. Before they could continue, they reached the rear entrance of the house. Reid held the door open and then followed Heather and Polaris inside.

"Have a seat at the table, Mr. Hunter. I'll have the coffee ready in a few minutes." As Reid sat at the wooden table, he watched Heather prepare the percolator. As she did, she continued to speak. "I've gone over your resume. You have a good work background and seem to be what I'm looking for. But I have one question that's been bothering me."

"Go ahead."

"Why didn't you wait for me to contact you after I'd received your resume?"

"Because I didn't want to wait in line," Reid responded truthfully. "There aren't very many jobs like this one available."

"I admire your initiative. How did you find out who placed the ad?" Reid told her of his ploy and listened as she laughed at his ingenuity. Then: "Why did you leave the Triple-K?"

"Kimball and I had a falling out. He owned the ranch and I left." Heather listened to every word he said, her senses alert to every nuance of his answer. Because of her blindness, Heather's other senses had developed keenly. She knew there was more to his answer, but also knew that what he said was true.

"If I decide to hire you, we can go into that a little further." Then, after pouring two cups of coffee, Heather began to interview Reid Hunter in earnest. She asked question after question, learning everything she could about this man, and when she was satisfied, she stopped.

"I can't give you an answer today, but if you'd like to

look around the ranch and see for yourself what we have, I'll have one of the men take you around."

"That would be fine," Reid said. Ten minutes later Reid was astride a roan gelding. He listened to what Tom Farley had to say and drank in every aspect of the ranch.

Chapter Two

Heather could not sit still. The incessant blaring of the radio kept breaking into her thoughts. She wanted quiet, a quiet that would permit her to think clearly. Suddenly she felt Polaris at her side and heard him bark, once.

"Go," she commanded in a low voice, "run." Polaris and she had been together for five years now. Her father had chosen the German shepherd puppy, the pick of the litter, and when he was a year old had taken him to a special school in Phoenix. Seven months later, Heather had both a companion and eyes, to replace the dog she had lost to old age. Polaris's commands were a little different from those of most seeing-eye dogs because he was a ranch dog, too. "Run," was his most-sought-after command. And it was only after dinner, when the ranch was quiet and Heather was in for the night, that Polaris was let free. Usually after an hour or two he came back. There was a special door in the kitchen wall that gave him free access. But Polaris never left Heather's side without her command. And Heather knew this no matter what Polaris did he was always near, always within hearing distance.

Heather listened to the padding of the shepherd's paws as he raced through the living room and into the kitchen. The telltale whoosh of his body as it brushed through the rubber barricade that opened like a tulip's petals told Heather Polaris was gone.

Moving slowly across the room, Heather reached for the stereo and shut it off. Then, with a sigh of contentment, she retraced the familiar path to the couch. After she sat, her fingers searched until they felt the hard plastic cassette, which she lifted and let her fingertips rub lightly across. In braille, she read the name.

Reid Hunter—Résumé

Quickly and efficiently, Heather placed the cassette into her tape player and placed her finger on the play button.

Ever since this morning's meeting with the man, her mind had been filled with thoughts of Reid Hunter. Her reaction to his voice, and even to the two times she had shaken his hand, had stirred feelings and emotions she had never known.

Desperately, since it had happened only a few rare times in her life, Heather wanted to see Reid Hunter's face. A ragged pain tore through her mind at this thought and tears began to rise.

"No!" she shouted to the empty house.

But her tears would not be denied. Heather found herself unable to stop them. *Why do I want so much?*

she asked herself. *Why? A blade of grass, that's all I want, to see a blade of grass. Oh, I can tell what a blade of grass looks like; I can tell its texture, its shape, even where the color changes from dark to lighter. I can sculpt it perfectly, I could even paint it if I had to, but I can't see it!*

Finally, after the tears stopped, Heather took a deep, cleansing breath and tried to relax. She hated feeling sorry for herself, hated the helpless and hopeless desire for what she knew was impossible. She'd lived for twenty-five years without her sight, and she knew she would live for a lot longer the same way. Heather did not usually permit herself the luxury of feeling sorry for herself, although there had been a time when she had. Now, except for occasional lapses of frustration, she had herself under iron control and enjoyed her life.

But Heather also knew that to cut off her thoughts and sorrows at this point would only bring them out again when she did not want them. She allowed her mind to wander and dwell on whatever memories it chose, knowing that doing so would help ease her hurt. This had been a trick her father had taught her years ago, when he was suffering his own losses.

Her father, Donald Strand, had been one of the two most important people in the world to Heather. He had been the mainstay of her life. Heather had been born blind, and she had never once seen the light of day. Her earliest memories were of her parents' voices and touches—holding her, carrying her, and putting her down so she could play on the grass. As she grew older, all of her senses grew with her. She learned how to see through her fingers and how to hear with her mind as well as her ears. When Heather was four, she had felt a growing distance between herself and her mother, a distance that did not foresake love, but one that forced her to rely on her father more and more.

When she was seven, her father had taken her onto his lap one day. She remembered that day clearly, sitting on his thighs, her head resting on his shoulders as he began to talk to her. His voice was different than usual; it held something she'd never heard before and was unable to identify. By the time he'd spoken his second sentence, Heather's fingers were tracing his face. It was then she'd felt the tears.

"I don't know exactly how to explain this, but I must," he said in a choked voice.

"Why are you sad, Daddy?" Heather asked.

"Heather, you're only seven years old. You're still a baby, but you're the bravest girl I ever knew." Heather heard a warm laugh build within his chest and felt her father's arm tighten around her even more. "Do you remember the time—I guess you were all of four—when you managed to get on my horse?"

"You spanked me!" Heather said indignantly.

"Yes, baby, I spanked you. But you wanted to ride, and you got on that horse. Didn't make any difference to you that you couldn't see where you were going—you just wanted to ride. . . ."

"I did good, didn't I?" Heather asked proudly.

"You sure did. . . ." Then Heather heard the change in his voice again and felt herself grow sad along with him. "Heather Jane Strand, I've got to tell you something. Your mama, she's very sick."

"Why are you sad? Mama's been sick before, just like me. You took good care of her," she told him matter-of-factly.

"This is different, girl. Your mama isn't going to get any better." Heather could tell by the way her father's chest rose and fell that he was badly upset, and because of that she was also.

"You mean Mama's always gonna be sick?"

"No, baby, she's not always going to be sick. Your mama . . ." he began, but paused for a deep breath. "Your mama's dying."

Heather knew what dying was. Puppet, her first seeing-eye dog, had died. Puppet had always slept with Heather; she'd been a soft, warm golden retriever. One morning Heather woke up, but no matter what she did, she couldn't get Puppet to move. Almost hysterical, she had called her mother. When her mother had come, she took Heather from the room and, in the kitchen, told her what had happened. Heather hadn't really understood right away, but eventually she had.

"Why, Daddy?" she asked, but this time her voice, too, sounded choked.

"Because no one can live forever. Sometimes people get very sick, and they die before we want them to. No one knows why—it just happens. It's happening to your mama, and you must try to understand."

Heather began to cry then, and Donald Strand pulled his little girl closer. He held her, and he cried with her, until finally Heather pulled away from him and slipped to the floor.

"Comet!" she called. A large German shepherd that came almost to Heather's shoulders moved next to the girl. Heather gripped the dog's collar. "Outside," she commanded.

Donald Strand watched his daughter, with her shoulders pulled back and her head held straight, walk from the house.

An hour later Heather returned. Her father was still sitting in the same chair, but she continued through the room and went into her parents' bedroom. At the door she told Comet to wait. Then, slowly, Heather made her way to the bed.

"Mama?" she called in a quiet voice.

"Yes, Heather?" her mother responded. Heather smiled at the soft sound of Justine Strand's voice and felt warmth and comfort flow through her.

"Can I talk to you?"

"Of course you can. Come sit on the bed next to me." Heather heard her pat the mattress as she walked toward the bed. Then she felt her mother's hands at her waist, helping her onto the bed, and noticed the weakness in them. Heather scooted closer to her mother, and her hands began to move by themselves. Her fingers traced the familiar paths of her mother's features, and as she touched the softness of her lips, she thought they felt the same as they always did. Her mother's cheeks were warm, warmer than usual, but they felt good, too. Then her small fingertips traced the eyebrows, the small straight nose, and began to stroke her hair. Suddenly Heather was crying, and uncontrollable sobs were torn from her throat.

"Easy, baby, you just take it easy," her mother cooed.

"Why, Mama, why?"

"I can't answer that, Heather. You know we always told each other the truth, and I won't lie to you now. I don't know why I'm sick. What I have is called cancer, and it's something the doctors don't know how to cure."

"Like me being blind?"

"Like your blindness," her mother agreed.

"But you don't feel any different," Heather told her.

"On the outside, no, but inside I'm real sick. Heather, Daddy told you what will happen to me, but you have to promise me something." Heather wiped away

26

her tears and nodded her head. "You've got to promise me that you'll take good care of your daddy when I'm gone."

"I don't want you to go!"

"I have to, baby. Promise?"

"I promise," Heather said reluctantly. After she said it, Heather lay down next to her mother, letting her mother hold her while she rested her head on the softness of her mother's breasts. Without realizing it, Heather fell asleep.

Years later Heather understood that her mother had purposely stayed a little distant during the last few years of her life to help ease the separation she knew was inevitable. Heather also learned that her mother had been sick for over three years.

Her mother died a month later, and Heather remembered her promise. She tried to take care of her father and her father had let her. When she was old enough to reason it out, she understood that her father had let her learn to cook and clean and do many of the things that most people do for two reasons. The first was to make her feel she was doing what her mother wanted; the second was so she would be able to grow up to lead a normal life.

As a child, Heather had always had a tutor. She had learned the braille alphabet by the time she was five. From age five until her mother died, she had another private tutor, who kept her at her level at grade school. But the fall after her mother died was the year her father sent her to a special school for the blind. There, with other blind children, she began to develop intellectually and socially. She came home for every vacation and each summer.

By the time she was in high school, she had talked her father into letting her live at home and attend the local public school. After the initial shock, Heather made herself fit in with the majority of the student body.

Along with high school came something else— something special. In the school for the blind art classes had been fun; it was the place where all the students had been encouraged to play and experiment. In high school art class became Heather's life. The teacher, Mr. Morrissey, had recognized something in Heather that no one else ever had. He had worked with her to bring it out, and Heather, in turn, had found something that grabbed her mind, her soul, and her heart, and held on like nothing else.

Art became the most important part of her life. There was only enough time for academics, her father, and her art. Nothing else was allowed to intrude. At first, she'd used ordinary soft modeling clay, and then Mr. Morrissey would make a mold and cast it in plaster. But by her senior year in high school Heather had reached the point of working with both stone and clay. By then she'd also begun to work on abstracts. Her father encouraged her every effort, and he, with several of his ranch hands, had built her a studio behind the house.

There had been little time in Heather's short life for dating and in that area Heather was almost ignorant. What she did know was that she did not enjoy the attention of the local boys. The one time she'd gone out with a boy in high school, it had been a disaster— nothing like what she'd read about in her books or listened to on her records.

The boy, Howie Conners, had stupidly taken her to a movie. But worse was when he had tried to explain what was happening on the screen. Heather had been amused at first, but as the movie went on she'd become impatient and then embarrassed as everyone kept shushing them. Finally, fighting back her tears, she asked Howie to take her home.

She didn't date again until college, and then went out only with other art majors. Most of the artists were understanding and knowledgeable about her blindness, and they were able to think in more than one dimension. She enjoyed her dates and had fun for the first time outside her family and her art. Then, in her junior year at Arizona State, she'd fallen in love. Or at least she thought she had.

Jim was tall and thin and had the most interesting facial structure she'd ever known. His lips were firm, and he had a thin mustache that reached to just the outer edge of his lip. He had blond hair that felt like the finest bristles of a perfect paintbrush, and he had large, doleful eyes. She knew how large they were because of the times she had traced them, but it was her roommate who told her how doleful they were. "Artist's eyes— large, sad, and longing."

She and Jim had dated on and off for the entire year, and finally, in her senior year, she admitted she was in love. And she truly thought she was. Heather had never had a real romance, or even something close to it. The hours and days she spent with Jim were like nothing else in her life. Soon they were kissing ardently and declaring their eternal love for each other. Then one night Heather gave herself to him. She had expected so much and had received so little. She'd even lost Jim. For three days after they had made love she did not hear from him. Then, on the fourth day, he came to her room. She heard it in his voice before he spoke three words.

"Why?" Heather demanded, cutting him off.

"I'm just sorry. I thought I loved you. I really did. . . ."

"But?"

"But after we . . . we made love, I felt terrible. It was like I seduced you and you couldn't see what I was doing. You would never see what I was like or what I looked like . . . or what I . . ."

"Stop it! You're not feeling guilty because you seduced a virgin, but because you think that my blindness stops me from being normal. That's it, isn't it? It doesn't make any difference to you that I know what you look like, that I can see you with my hands and within my mind. I know every line of your face, of your body, better than anyone with sight! But it's only that I can't see you that matters."

"Heather, no, it's . . ."

"Get out!" Heather ordered. She hoped he would fight, that he would tell her she was wrong and ask to stay. But, silent as the night, Jim left.

Heather broke down after that and cried until dawn. When she woke the next morning, it was to her promise that no one would ever get that close to her heart again. And it had been just that way. She had her father, and that was enough.

It was enough until two years ago, when her father had been killed in a freak accident. Donald Strand had been driving into town one afternoon when a young boy who had lost control of his pony galloped onto the highway. Her father had been driving at about fifty miles an hour when the boy appeared in front of him. Donald Strand turned the steering wheel hard to avoid hitting the youth and had run off the road and into a tree. He'd hit his head on the steering wheel and never awakened. His skull had been fractured. Heather's father had died before he reached the hospital.

Since then Heather had been running the ranch, to the sacrifice of her art. It was not something she took lightly, nor did she regret what she had to give up. This was her home, as it had been her mother's and father's. Without the Strand Ranch, there could be no Heather, and no art.

By the time things had settled down and the ranch was back to normal, Heather had made peace with herself over her father's death. For the next four months Heather worked with the foreman, Hank Thompson, learning everything she had not bothered with until then. Her mind opened and she learned what was necessary to run a ranch. A year later, Hank gave notice. Heather was torn, not knowing what to do. Hank had been offered a good job with a much larger ranch and a lot more money. Heather did not try to talk him out of it: he had children and a wife to support. With her approval, Hank Thompson left.

Then Heather had talked Tom Farley into taking over as the foreman. Tom had tried, but even Heather knew he was not experienced enough to handle the job. Reluctantly she agreed with Tom and began to advertise. The first time there were a dozen responses, each falling into two categories.

There were those in whom she sensed a hesitancy in their manner about working not only for a woman, but a blind woman. Those men she ruled out immediately. Then came the other types—the ones who seemed to be itching for the job. Heather knew they would use the ranch, and her, to do whatever they wanted. These, too, she dismissed out of hand.

Then she advertised again. This time there had been

ten responses. Out of the ten, three seemed to be good possibilities. Of the three, only two had prior experience as a foreman. Today she had spoken with Reid Hunter; on Tuesday she would interview John Scotts.

As Heather's mind returned to the present, she let out a sigh. She knew she could not be weak in front of people, especially those who worked for her, and had found, during these last two years without her father to talk to, that these little trips into the past seemed to help more than hurt. They helped her survive and made her stronger.

Gently, Heather pressed the play button on the recorder and began to listen to Emma Kline's voice as she dictated Reid Hunter's resume for Heather to listen to. This would be the third time she'd heard it and the first time she would be able to match the resume with the man.

Emma's clear diction and low but distinct voice called for Heather's attention.

"'Reid Hunter. Age, thirty-four. Height, six feet, one-half inch. Weight, one hundred eighty-five pounds.'"

Then there was the barest of pauses as Emma said, "He's a real hunk, Heather—at least on paper." This was followed by a little giggle before Emma began to speak in a serious voice again.

"'Eyes, Hazel. Hair, Brown. Born, Lander, Wyoming. Education, public high school, University of Wyoming. Employment. First job, G-bar-D ranch, Boise, Wyoming, five years. Army, Vietnam. Honorable discharge. Assistant Foreman, Pegasus Ranch, Butte, Montana, four years. Triple-K Ranch, Phoenix, Arizona, two years. Reason for leaving, personal.'

—Aren't they all?" Emma's taped voice commented. "That's it on this one. No picture."

Heather turned off the recorder, entwined her fingers together, and rested her chin on their backs. *Personal reasons . . . yes,* thought Heather, *a man like Reid Hunter would have strong feelings.* But somewhere in the back of her mind a thought rose. Reid Hunter had a better work record than most cowboys in their twenties and thirties, and Heather realized that Reid Hunter's reason for leaving the Triple-K would be one of his own moral code, not what the rest of the world would consider a good reason.

Cowboys were different from other men—no matter if they were educated and held a Master of Business Administration degree—they were still cowboys; they were a breed apart.

A light tapping at the front door pulled Heather's mind from her thoughts. "Open," she called. She heard the door open and heard footsteps come into the living room. "Evening, Tom," she said as she recognized the special pattern of footfalls that told her who he was.

"Evening, Heather. You said you wanted to speak to me tonight?"

"Have a seat." While she waited for Tom to sit and stretch out his long legs, she formulated exactly what she wanted to say. Tom was her right-hand man, a man whose instincts she trusted implicitly.

"I want your feelings, your deep-down gut reactions to Reid Hunter," she said to him.

The music from the jukebox beat a steady tattoo inside Reid Hunter's head. But he ignored it, as he had for ten years. He lifted his beer and sipped it. He didn't want to be here, sitting at a back table in a two-bit honky-tonk on the outskirts of Tahoe, but it was better than sitting alone in his room. Usually it didn't matter if he was alone—most of the time he preferred it—but not today. At least this place had people in it. Live people, not the plastic executives who pretended to be alive so they could get a name put on their dotted lines and throw their money away on the crap tables. Here, Reid felt as if he blended, even though he didn't. The old bar had once been a light wood, but now looked old, stained, and comfortable. The bartender looked like an old cowboy who had busted one bronc too many at the local rodeo and ended up behind the bar instead of throwing his prize money across it.

The walls were decorated with rodeo posters, and Reid knew every name on them. The crowd was thin—the usual Sunday-night people, he thought. There were maybe a dozen men in the place and half that number of women. Everyone was low-key, maybe because of the hour or because they'd all be getting up early the next morning.

Reid pulled his eyes from the people and stared at his beer bottle. Since he'd left the Strand ranch, he'd been unable to get Heather Strand out of his mind. He thought about her again—about her beauty and about his own reaction when he'd discovered her blindness.

At first, he'd felt sad—not the pity she'd accused him of, but just a sadness for someone who could not see what was around them. But, as he'd listened to her talk, he'd realized that she was able to see in her own way and the sadness had left him. But he was still bothered. He didn't have the same prejudices about women that most ranchmen had, but all the same, he knew that working for a woman boss was not the easiest thing in the world.

A blind woman. That would be even harder. Reid

wanted to know how she had lost her sight, or at least when. He didn't know why, but it was constantly on his mind. He also wanted the job—more now than before, and before he had wanted it badly.

Then his mind skipped back to Arizona and the Triple-K Ranch, where he'd been the foreman and loved it. He'd done his job well, and it showed. After the first year, Reid had started to change things. Slowly, he figured. Do it slowly and do it right. The first few things he'd done worked beautifully, and even Kingston had told him so. Rafe Kingston was a legend in ranching, and for him to compliment anyone was an accomplishment. Foremen came and went at the Triple-K as fast as a thunderstorm in the mountains.

But three months ago trouble had started. The trouble was Kelly Kingston. Kelly was Rafe's daughter, twenty-one years old and ready to prowl. Kelly had red hair and gray eyes. She was five feet, six inches of perfectly formed flesh and bones, and she knew it. So had Reid, and he hadn't wanted any part of it.

Reid shook his head to clear the memories, but the cool gray eyes stayed in his mind. Lifting the bottle, Reid took another pull of the cold beer. As he did, he felt someone come up behind him. He put the bottle down slowly and turned.

"Hunter? Reid Hunter, you old bastard!" said the burly cowboy who stood above him. "Heard you were 'the man' at the Triple-K."

"Evenin', Steve," Reid said in a cool voice as he looked the man over.

"What the hell are you doin' in Tahoe?"

"Having a beer."

"Jesus, Reid, what's it been—six years?" asked Steve Higgins.

"Must be," replied Reid as he stood up. "Don't

mean to be impolite, but I've got to get up early. See you around," he said as he gave the cowboy a half-smile and started away.

"Same old hard-assed bastard as always, aren't you, Hunter?"

"I guess so," Reid replied as he walked out of the bar.

"Damn," murmured the burly cowboy as he watched Reid leave. "I never believed them rumors, but maybe they're true. . . ."

Chapter Three

*T*hen you agree?" Heather asked Tom Farley. They were seated in the ranch office, in Heather's father's office, with Heather behind the large desk and Tom seated across from her. They could both hear the typewriter beating steadily as Emma Kline worked up her monthly report.

"Between Hunter and the other man there's no choice. Emma's checked him out with the Triple-K people and they've verified his employment. Good recommendation," Tom Farley declared.

"You think you'll be comfortable as his assistant?"

"From the time I spent with him on Sunday and the questions he asked, yes."

"Okay, Tom. I'll call him," Heather said. Tom stood, knowing their business was finished and that he had work to do. Before he reached the door, Heather called out to him. "Seeing anyone yet?"

"No one special, Heather," he replied. Heather caught the underlying sadness in his voice, but refrained from saying anything.

"That pony about ready for Gregg?"

"He's ready," Tom replied as he opened the office door.

"Emma will have the figures tonight. Come by after Gregg's asleep and we'll go over them if you're up to it."

"I'll be by about nine," Tom told her as he walked from the office, leaving the office door open.

"Emma," Heather called, "try getting Reid Hunter on the phone. Have him meet me for lunch tomorrow at the Pine Tree."

"Yes, ma'am," Emma called in her cheerful voice.

Heather smiled. Emma Kline had been her father's bookkeeper for almost fifteen years. When he had died, Heather had made Emma promise to stay on and to not only be the ranch bookkeeper, but to act as her assistant as well. Emma was known as the local spinster, but Heather knew it had been by choice. There had been someone years ago who had won Emma's heart, but something had happened to him and Emma had never had the desire for another man.

Heather sniffed the air. The day was dry and comfortable, and the scents of pine mixed with soil filled her senses and brought a smile to her lips. Suddenly the smile disappeared from her mouth as she thought about Tom and Gregg Farley. Tom had come to work at the ranch when Heather was in her last year of college. She remembered being introduced to Tom and three-year-old Gregg five years ago.

Heather's father had told her that one night Tom had knocked on the door seeking shelter for himself and his young son when their car had broken down. Donald Strand had taken them in, and the next day he had learned the tall man's story.

Tom had been working for a bank in Carson City as a loan officer. One night he had come home to find his son with a baby-sitter and a note from his wife. She had left them. Tom, for some reason, decided to leave the small apartment they had lived in and drive to California. The old car had not made it, and Tom had ended up at the Strand Ranch.

Donald Strand had offered Tom a job, even though he'd never worked a ranch before. Tom accepted the job and the small house for himself and Gregg. Ever since then he'd applied himself to learning how to work a ranch and had found he had a natural ability for the work. In the five years he'd been there, Tom had become a strong, independent man who loved what he did and loved his son just as much.

Heather also knew it had taken Tom a long time to get over his wife's desertion, although nobody could tell by his face or his actions. But Heather knew it was time for him to be seeing other women; Gregg needed a mother and Tom needed a woman who cared for him.

"All set," called Emma, pulling Heather from her thoughts. "One o'clock."

"Thank you, Emma. The only other thing I'll need before you leave is the monthly figures."

"Almost finished," replied Emma.

"Good," Heather responded.

"Not really, hon. Sorry," Emma said in a lower voice.

"I knew that already," Heather whispered. "Reid Hunter, you'd better be what I need!" she said under her breath. Heather knew that the ranch would be in trouble if things weren't straightened out soon. But she also knew, after two days of deep thought, that she, too, might be in trouble—in trouble because of the way her mind was going on about Reid Hunter.

The first pinkish gray bands of light began to filter through the bamboo thicket. The smells of decay, rotting vegetation, and human filth filled Lieutenant Reid Hunter's nostrils. He, his commanding officer, and the platoon had been on a search-and-destroy mission for ten days. Below them was the next village. In the ten days he'd been in the jungle, Reid had lost seven of the thirty men he'd started with—five in firefights, one to a sniper, and another to a Cong booby trap. Framed neatly in his field glasses, he saw the village begin to come to life. Children and women came from their huts, some to start the cooking fires, others to bring water.

Damn! thought Reid, *not one man.* Where were they? Reid had seen dozens of villages like this one, devoid of men and boys over eleven. The Cong had come and taken them to fight on their side. The villagers had no choice. Reid had also seen villages that seemed like this one until they got within rifle distance. Then he found himself in a nightmare world of careening bullets from the hidden Cong in the huts and in the tunnels that were like mazes beneath the villages.

"Let's get ready, Hunter," ordered Captain Aaron Fielding. Reid fought away his initial anger at the man's voice. Fielding was on his first long patrol and he was the general's hotshot new boy! He was interested in only two things, body counts and glory.

"Sir, I'd like to hold off for a little while. Let's see if there are any men down there."

"I said to get the platoon ready. If there are any men there, they're Charlie, and they're hiding."

"Sir," Reid argued.

"Move it, Lieutenant!"

"Yes, sir!" Reid said as he turned and went back to his men. He didn't like the feelings that flowed through him, about the captain and about the village. Reid moved through his men, his sergeant at his side, as he gave the men their orders. Five minutes later, they started down the hill. Reid and a corporal named Trigent, who spoke fluent Vietnamese, held the point. Reid wouldn't stay in the main body—he wasn't one to let his men take anything for him.

Slowly they walked into the village. The women and children stopped what they were doing and watched the American soldiers come toward them. Reid felt his pulse racing, tasted the fear that rose up in his mouth, but stood tall, holding the M-16 in front of him and keeping a shallow smile on his face.

They reached the center of the village and stopped. "Trigent, start your spiel," Reid ordered.

Trigent began to speak in the dialect of the area, and as he did, the rest of the platoon began to walk into the village. Reid made a mistake then—he began to relax as his eyes turned back to his men. It was only for a fraction of a second, but it was long enough.

Suddenly he heard Trigent hesitate. Reid felt the hair at the nape of his neck stand out and whirled just as the shot rang out. Reid felt the corporal's body hit him, knocked back by the impact of the bullet. Falling to the ground, Reid brought his rifle to the ready position as the bullets from his own men flew over his head. The firing stopped before Reid had fired a single shot.

Reid stood and looked at the dead enemy. His eyes

went wide in shock. Then, violently, wave after wave of sickness rushed through his body.

"No!" The single word seemed to pull Reid from his nightmare. He felt the coolness of the air conditioning against his naked body, felt the perspiration that glistened on his body, and realized where he was.

On and off for ten years, Reid Hunter had had the same nightmare. In the first years following his return home they had come nightly. Now they came infrequently. But when they did, it was bad. Reid threw the sheet from his body and stood. He began to pace his motel room, trying to shake the tenseness that filled him. The feeling of horror and defeat still held him in thrall. *Will I ever stop dreaming it?* he asked himself. *Ten years of running, of trying to live with myself, of trying to find myself. Ten years and it's still the same.*

"Think of something else!" he ordered himself in a husky voice. Then he stopped and shook his head. He had a lunch date with Heather Strand in . . . Reid turned on the small table lamp and looked at his watch—5:00 A.M.—eight hours.

A picture of Heather rose in Reid's mind. The soft brown hair, pretty blue eyes, and perfectly formed face floated within the confines of his mind. Reid thought about their lunch date today. Would she ask any more questions about the Triple-K? If she did, would he tell her about Kingston's daughter and the real reason he'd left? Or had she checked out his whole resume? Had she found out his lies of the early years of his past and his real heritage? *No. If she had, she wouldn't be meeting me today,* he thought.

Reid reached for the pack of cigarillos that were on the nightstand. He pulled one from the pack and lit it quickly. Inhaling the acrid smoke, Reid began to force himself to relax. As the smoke drifted upward, playing a lazy pattern within the lamplight, he began to think about the dream again.

When he was discharged from the army and had returned to civilian life, Reid found that he no longer cared for what was his. The only thing that mattered was his being able to try to live with what he'd done and make a new life for himself. He'd arrived home, in Albuquerque, to the joy of his sister and brother, but soon they, too, discovered Reid Hunter was a far different man than he'd been before he left.

Patrick Hunter had expected his brother to come back to the ranch and run it with him. He'd expected Reid to put the college education he'd completed during the four years previous to joining the army to good use at their ranch. Their father had died five years before and he'd left the ranch to his sons, Reid and Patrick, and to his daughter Gwen. But Reid had stayed only long enough to get his old clothes, buy a car, and sign over his rights to the ranch by giving Patrick full power of attorney. Then he said good-bye to the two people who loved but did not understand him and started the life of a homeless cowboy.

"You can't do this to us!" Pat Hunter had flared in anger. "You can't walk out on us. We need you here."

"You're doing just fine, both of you," Reid told them. Gwen cried, unashamedly letting her tears fall. She knew what had happened, to a degree, and was both hurt and frightened for Reid. But Pat was a different story. Reid had not shared what had happened to him with his brother. He knew that Pat would not understand. The enemy was the enemy—period! So Reid had left Broadlands, the ninety-thousand-acre ranch that his great-grandfather had built, put behind him the life of power, wealth, and family in order to retrieve what he had lost in Vietnam—himself.

Reid had had plenty of money. Each of the three children had received substantial inheritances from their father along with a third ownership in the ranch. After Reid had given over his power of attorney to Patrick, he took his large inheritance and donated it to a charity he had helped form.

A lot had happened during the last ten years—a lot and nothing at all. His sister, Gwen, had left the ranch six years ago to open a small business of her own in Santa Fe. She left bitterly, also at odds with Patrick because of what he'd done to her. She had fallen in love with one of her college professors and Patrick had not approved. Patrick had forced an end to the affair and Gwen had felt she had no choice but to leave, bury the past, and start anew.

For Reid it wasn't that simple. He was still plagued by his past, and nothing seemed to rid him of it. Even Sunday night, when he was at that honky-tonk bar and Steve Higgins had come in, his past had come with it. Steve had known Reid when he first started out from New Mexico, had worked with him both at his own ranch and at the first job he'd taken. Reid had lied about his work background, and when the foreman heard what Higgins was telling the others, he'd called Reid into his office and talked to him. The foreman thought Reid was out to steal ideas or some nonsense like that. Reid had told him that he'd left the ranch and just wanted to work. The foreman seemed to have understood him and let him stay on. Reid had taken Steve Higgins aside and told him that if he ever repeated Reid's background he would break him in half. He never had to; Higgins saw too much in Reid's eyes to take the chance.

What was Higgins doing in Nevada? Reid wondered about the cowboy and hoped like hell he wasn't working at the Strand Ranch.

With that thought Reid crushed out the thin cigarillo, stretched, and went back to bed. He knew he would sleep undisturbed for however long he wanted to. That was something else he had learned. When he had his dream, it happened only once in a night. Never twice.

Reid shut off the light, lay down in bed, and willed the sleep to overtake him.

Heather stepped from the shower, letting the water cascade from her body. She felt good; she always did after a shower. She reached for a towel, bent her head over, and wrapped her hair within it. When the turban was finished, she reached for the heavier terry cloth bath towel and began to massage herself dry.

When Heather was satisfied that every inch of her skin was dry, she powdered herself with Ciara, enjoying the fresh, clean smell of the perfumed powder and the refreshing feel of it on her skin. Then she went into her bedroom and to her dresser. Carefully her fingers searched through the drawer until they found what she wanted. Her lightweight bra with its matching lace panties were withdrawn. Heather slipped her arms through the straps of the front-closing bra. Leaning forward, she let her firm breasts fill the cups as she closed the bra. Then she slipped the panties on and adjusted them over her hips. When she wasn't wearing jeans and men's shirts, Heather enjoyed the feel of soft and silky clothing against her skin. She enjoyed it almost as much as when she sculpted.

Heather stood in the bedroom debating over what she should wear. With a quick smile and nod to herself, she turned back to the dresser and withdrew a silk half-slip. After this was on, Heather returned to the bathroom, undid the towel on her hair, and began to blow the hair dry. She used her fingers, letting the warm air of the dryer flow through her hair and hands. Her natural waves would take over by the time her hair was dry, and only a few quick brushstrokes would be needed to control it. Heather liked her hair to fall naturally. It wasn't vanity—it just felt good to her that way.

At the closet Heather hesitated. At first she'd considered wearing a suit in order to be businesslike. But now she was unsure. She didn't dress up very often, and she hated to make all her effort go to waste.

Letting her fingers run along the clothes rack, Heather felt for each item. Above each hanger was a braille code letter to tell her the color of the item. Three times Heather stopped and felt an article of clothing. Three times Heather rejected it. Then Heather's fingers touched another code letter and her hands went to the dress. She nodded again and pulled it free.

This dress was a cinnamon color with a button-down front and a lace collar. It had a wide belt and a nicely pleated skirt. The hem of the dress fell midway between her knee and calf. Heather stepped into the dress, buttoned it, and then belted it. She let her hands run along her sides, roll over her hips, and then smooth out the flare of the skirt. She did the same thing along her derrière and over her stomach and breasts.

The material, sheer to the touch, but opaque, felt pleasantly soft against the palms of her hands. Heather knew she would not be overdressed for her luncheon interview, but would stand out amongst the crowd.

Heather laughed. Polaris would stand out anywhere. Heather knew that no matter what she wore her dog would cause everyone's eyes to follow her if she brought him with her. She went back to the closet and found the matching shoes. The shoes had a small gold strap across the front and medium heels. Heather slipped into the shoes and left the bedroom. At the front door she called Polaris, who accompanied her to the office.

"Aren't we the pretty one," stated Emma as Heather entered.

"Do I look all right?" Heather asked as she executed a pirouette before Emma.

"Gorgeous! Oh . . ."

"What?" Heather asked, alarmed.

"Your shoes. They're green."

"Oh, no," Heather cried. "Gregg promised he'd stop tricking me if I gave him a paying chore. I'm going to get that little devil . . ." Heather declared as she started to turn and go back to her house.

"Hold it, turkey, I'm only kidding." At the relief Emma saw in Heather's face, she began to laugh softly. "Got ya!"

"One day I'm going to get even," Heather swore, but she smiled as she said it.

"Are you ready?" Emma asked.

"As ready as ever. I do hope Reid Hunter needs this job badly. Especially for what we're going to pay him."

"Tell him you'll cook dinner every night—maybe that'll persuade him," Emma offered good-naturedly. "Come on, let's get you over to the restaurant."

Chapter Four

Heather stepped into the bathtub for the second time today, but this time she sank gratefully into its warmth. She felt the hot water cover her and let herself be caressed by it. After a moment, she laid her head against the porcelain and began to breathe softly.

She ran her hands along her legs, feeling the firmness of her skin and muscles. She traced them as an artist would, with her mind on their lines. Her calves were smooth, lean, and she knew their shape was almost perfect. Her thighs were firm and the warm skin on them was smooth. Her hands and fingers rose along her hips, and there, too, she felt the firmness of her skin and muscles. Her fingers skimmed across her flat stomach, over the muscles that lay just below the skin. Her hands rose to her breasts and felt them critically. They were firm, not large, and the muscles that supported them held them high. Her neck was long—just a drop too long for a classic model—and it was one reason that Heather never had done a bust of herself. When she sculpted from a live model, especially a woman, there were certain things that she demanded as an artist. One was the correct proportions.

It was not the beauty of the person—not their actual physical beauty—but a beauty of proportion that Heather loved to work with. Like Gregg Farley. At eight years old, his proportions were magnificent. His neck, shoulders, and head were perfect. But, Heather conceded, even if they weren't, she would have done a bust of Gregg anyway. His mind and his whole being were beautiful.

Heather shook away the thoughts of her art as she reached for the bar of soap. Gently, enjoying the luxurious vanity and the needed relaxation of this bath, she began to wash herself. In Heather's world everything was touch, sound, or scent, and for Heather the feel of the gentle soap rubbing along her skin with the soft terry washcloth was almost like heaven.

When she finished washing, she pulled the drain and the soapy water began to run out. When the water was more than half gone, Heather closed the drain and began to run fresh water into the bath. When it was again filled with the hot water, she put her arms on the sides of the tub and let her head sink slowly back as her mind began to wander to today's lunch with Reid Hunter.

Emma had pulled the car to a stop at the front entrance of the restaurant. The Pine Tree was one of the oldest restaurants in the area, and Heather Strand's most favorite. She had been going there since she was a child.

"You're sure you don't want me to stay? I can wait for you. Really, it's no problem," Emma said.

"No. Go have lunch and take care of those other matters in town. I should be ready in two hours," Heather said as the car door was opened by the attendant. Heather felt Polaris move and put her hand on his head. "Stay," she commanded him, deciding not to bring the dog inside the restaurant with her.

As Heather left the car, she felt the attendant's hand go to her arm. "Two steps, Miss Strand."

"My goodness, Chuck, after all these years don't you think I know how many steps there are?" she asked, and laughed lightly. "And after the two steps are six steps to the door, five steps in, and then turn left."

"Yes, ma'am," Chuck responded, and Heather heard the humor in his voice. She smiled at him and patted his hand.

"Thank you, Chuck," she said as he held the door open for her. By the time she passed through the door, every scent in the restaurant assaulted her. She could smell the beef roasting in the ovens, the vegetables that were steaming on the stoves, and the sweet scent of flowers on each table. The scent of gardenias stood out among them all. Then she smelled another scent, and her stomach growled in response. Brook trout—oh, how she loved fresh brook trout.

"Heather, hi, how are you?" asked a familiar voice.

"Caroline, it's been a while. I'm fine. Yourself, the boys?" she asked with a smile and an outstretched hand. Heather's hand was grasped by the other woman's.

"They're fine. It's good to see you. Why, it must be three months, and it's all my fault. I know I promised to call."

"I know how busy you are," Heather said graciously, excusing her friend from the lapse. Caroline Buckman and she had been friends since high school and kept in contact regularly. But, with Caroline's work at the restaurant and her two boys, their times together had become less and less frequent. "I'm meeting a Mr. Hunter for lunch. Is he here yet?"

"He sure is. Been here for about fifteen minutes. At your regular table," Caroline informed her.

"Thanks. I'll find my own way. Oh, the trout smells wonderful," she said as she began to walk toward her table. The table was the same one she always sat at and the most direct from the entrance. She knew exactly what the restaurant looked like, even though she'd never seen it. It was a large room with forty tables. Each table was set a small distance from its neighbors, comfortable, almost private, yet very open. The paintings on the walls had been done by local artists and were among the best in the state. Her table was set in the middle of a bank of windows against the left-hand wall of the restaurant and, Heather knew, it overlooked a small pond. The pond was surrounded by evergreens, and in spring and summer it was lush with flowers. There were several cement benches set near its edge, and dividing the benches was one of her own sculptures, an abstract she'd done a few years ago. As she walked and smelled the wonderful scents of the food and flowers, she felt at home.

Stopping exactly three feet from her table, Heather heard a chair scrape along the floor. "Good afternoon, Mr. Hunter," she said.

"Afternoon, ma'am," Reid replied. She could sense his movement as he came around the table and pulled out the chair for her. Then his hand was on her arm, guiding her to the chair. Again she felt that jolt of electricity from his fingers and her breath caught.

"Thank you," she finally said as she sat down. After he returned to his seat, Heather smiled. "Sorry to keep you waiting."

"I was early, you're on time," he informed her politely. "Would you like to order?"

"To be honest, the minute I stepped in here I became ravenous," she said. It was true, but her appetite had left her when he had touched her. *Why,* she wondered, *is he affecting me like this?*

"I . . . er . . . Damn! Sorry, but I don't know what I'm supposed to do. Do I read you the menu?" he asked.

A bubbly laugh rose in her throat. "In a place I'm not familiar with that would be appropriate, but I know the menu here by heart," she told him.

"I should have known that already," Reid said with a low laugh of his own. Then the waitress came. Both declined drinks and ordered their lunch. Heather chose trout and a small salad. Reid ordered the same. After the waitress left, Heather knew Reid was gazing at her. She waited for him to speak.

"Please don't take what I'm about to say in the wrong way," he began. Heather nodded. "You're a beautiful young woman, and a talented one too. Why are you trying to run the ranch? You could sell it and make enough to keep you in a nice way for a long time."

Heather felt herself grow angry and her muscles began to tense. Willfully, she forced herself to relax. "I thought I made that clear the other day, Mr. Hunter. This ranch has been in my family for a long time, and I plan on keeping it that way."

"I understand that. But you're . . ."

"I'm what," she demanded, forcing the man to put words to his thought.

"You're blind," he said simply.

"And?"

"And nothing. How can you run a ranch? How can you check on what's happening, see what your help is doing?"

"Trust, Mr. Hunter, trust."

"That's very risky," Reid told her bluntly.

"It's all I can do. That's why you're here."

"What happened to your last foreman?" he asked. Heather relaxed, the anger of a moment ago subsiding as she realized his questions had not been mocking, but honest and sincere.

"I'll have to start at the beginning." When she received no response, she began. "When my father died, Hank Thompson was the foreman. He stayed on for a year and taught me a lot, but then he received a better offer. I couldn't stop him—he's got a wife and two kids and he needed the extra money. Tom Farley took over then, but Tom doesn't want to be the foreman. He's been nice enough to handle everything until I hired the right man."

The waitress interrupted them with their food. As they ate, they talked about the area and about anything except the ranch. Throughout the meal Heather felt herself reacting to Reid's voice, his manner, and the way he spoke. Everything within her seemed primed to explode whenever he spoke, and the ability to use her willpower, the willpower that she had trained herself to achieve during her growing years, was never more strained than now. She didn't know what it was, this magnetism that radiated from Reid. But she fought it, and won, and nothing of her internal turmoil showed on her face. When they were finished with the meal, the dishes cleared and the coffee served, they began to talk once again about the ranch.

Reid took the initiative, throwing Heather off stride

until she realized what he was doing. When she understood, she let herself go, explaining every detail that Reid wanted to know. By the time he was finished, Heather knew that Reid Hunter was the man she needed to run the ranch.

"Have my references checked out okay?" he asked.

"They were fine," Heather said with a nod. Suddenly she needed to touch him, to feel his face, and to learn what he looked like. *But not here,* Heather thought, *not in the restaurant.* He was a cowboy, and she knew by the little time they had spoken that he was part of that breed who kept their emotions private, who showed no public displays. A woman touching a man's face in public, as she would have to do, might embarrass him.

"Mr. Hunter, will you tell me the reason you left the Triple-K? From what I learned Mr. Kingston respected and admired you. And from what I understand that doesn't happen too often with him." She heard Reid take in a breath, hold it for a moment, and then let it out slowly.

"Miss Heather, it really was a personal reason. It had nothing to do with my job," he told her. Heather knew he was speaking the truth.

"Mr. Hunter, when can you start?" Heather asked, her mind made up.

"When you start calling me Reid," he responded. Heather smiled and stretched out her hand. She felt Reid take it in his strong hand and clasp it tightly. She felt the dry warmth of his hand, the power and strength within it. They stayed like that for several seconds before Heather reluctantly withdrew her hand.

"Reid," she said, using his name for the first time, almost savoring it, "we haven't discussed salary or anything."

"I'm not worried. Whatever the last foreman was getting will be fine. Is that all right, Miss Heather?"

"It will be, if you'll call me Heather when you're not working." Heather waited, knowing that this was another form of the code. Women who were owners of ranches were always called *miss*, even though most foremen called their male bosses by the first name.

"When do I start . . . Heather?" Reid asked.

"When can you bring your things out and get settled?"

"Right after lunch," he told her, and Heather sensed the smile that was surely on his face.

The warmth of the water departed as her mind returned to the present, and Heather sat up. Not wanting to leave the bath yet, she again turned on the hot water. Two minutes later the bath was once more comfortable, and she lay back. Yes, she thought, she was glad she'd hired Reid Hunter. They'd even fought over the check. Reid had won, telling her that he wasn't working for her until he brought his things to the ranch, and had insisted on paying the check. When they were outside, Reid had asked how she was getting back to the ranch. She'd told him that someone was picking her up. Reid had told her that he was already checked out of the motel and would be going to the ranch today to settle in. Could he drive her home?

She agreed. Heather told Chuck, the attendant, that when Emma came for her to just send her on to the ranch.

They drove in silence until they neared the ranch. Although Reid started to tell her where they were, Heather had smiled and told him she knew. She could smell the familiar scent of her home.

"Pull over," she had ordered him suddenly. Reid had complied and then asked why.

"I've hired you, I've listened to you, and I know some of your background. Now I need to know what you look like," she had told him. As she had spoken, she'd felt her heart beating quickly within her. She could almost hear the staccato pounding deep within her chest and, as hard as she tried, she could not control it. Part of what she had said was the truth, but only part. She wanted to touch him, to know him as only a blind person could.

"I'm not sure what you mean," Reid had said to her.

"It's simple. Being blind doesn't mean I can't know what people or things look like. I use my fingers and hands for that. Like this," she had said as she had moved her hands toward his voice.

Heather had been afraid her hands were trembling but dredged up a last bit of willpower and forced them to be still. She had started at his chin, moving her fingers slowly, tracing the outline of his jaw. She felt the beginning of his beard's stubble, although she could also tell that he'd shaved that morning. He would have a strong beard; he'd probably have to shave twice a day if he were going out at night. Heather's fingers traced his jawline and her heart beat harder. Reid's jaw was smooth, strong, and angular, with the slightest of indentations near its center—a small cleft. Her fingers continued their course, tracing his cheeks. His cheek-bones were strong, well formed. Then her fingers had dipped to his lips—full lips, soft skin, not hard and chapped like so many outdoorsmen. Against her fingers she had felt his mustache and had traced its outline. The mustache had been thick, straight, but not wiry. She had felt his even breathing, warm wisps that came from his nose and flowed across her fingers. Then, slowly, she had traced his nose. Not too large, almost straight. She knew that it would look straight, but there was a slight bump in the middle.

"Broken?" she had asked.

"When I was ten," Reid had replied, and she had felt the skin of his face pull tight in a smile. "Most people can't tell," he told her.

She had smiled as her fingers moved on. She wasn't most people. She had traced his large eyes. His eyebrows had been thick, but not broad. Reid's ears were in perfect proportion to his face and almost hugged his head. Her fingers found the indentations near his eyes and knew the crow's-feet would only add grace and character to his face. Finally, she had traced his forehead, feeling the broadness of it, and the grooves that ran across it. From squinting in the sun, she had thought.

"Do you approve?" he had asked, but Heather had been able to tell from his voice that the question had been anything but lightly asked.

"You're a handsome man, Reid Hunter. You've got a strong face, a face that most people would trust. I approve," she had said at last, smiling as she had tried to hide the heaviness of her own emotion. "If you want to go on, I'm ready now."

"I . . ."

There had been a long silence then, until Heather had realized exactly what she had said. The tension flew from her and from the inside of the vehicle. She laughed at the sudden thought that had flashed in her mind and said, "To the ranch."

"Yes, ma'am," Reid had replied as he shifted the Land-Rover into gear and started back onto the road.

He was handsome. His face was strong, clean of line, not pretty, not soft, but held a strong masculinity and self-assurance. Again Heather realized that she had hired the right man.

With that thought, Heather finally stood and opened the drain. At the same time, she tried to calm the aching within her. Stepping from the tub, she wrapped herself in a terry towel. Five minutes later she was in her nightgown, with a robe over it. She left the bathroom and went into the kitchen. There she put water into the teakettle and placed the kettle on the fire.

Polaris came next to her and pressed against her leg. She bent, letting her fingers glide along his back. Turning, Heather lifted her hands to her chest and patted twice. "Give a hug," she told the dog. Suddenly the large shepherd rose on his hind legs, his front paws gently falling on her shoulders as he stretched his neck to place his muzzle against the side of her cheek. Heather sensed the affection from the dog; his love and obedience made her feel warm. Her hands rubbed briskly along his fur for a moment before releasing him.

"Good boy," she said. "Okay, Polaris, run!" The dog barked once. Then she heard him walk to his door and slip through to freedom. The whistle from the kettle sounded and Heather pulled it from the fire and got a cup and teabag. She poured the water into the cup and smelled the tangy scent of the English tea. With a smile Heather took the cup and sat at the kitchen table, listening to the night sounds of the Strand Ranch and wondering if Reid was settling in comfortably.

Chapter Five

April flowed quietly into May; May blended into June. With the heat of the early summer day filling the air around her, Heather paused at her work. Her ears had picked up footsteps, and when they stopped, so had she.

She heard Polaris get up from the floor and make his way softly toward the door. "Hey, boy," came Reid's voice and the sound of his hand scratching the shepherd. Probably behind his ear, Heather thought. Despite the heat in the studio, a curious chill ran along her spine. It was almost as if it were she who Reid had touched rather than the dog. The first thing Heather did was put a damp towel over the clay, then her fingers went to her wrist. She traced the time on the watch—three o'clock.

"No problems," Reid said as he saw her gesture. "I just wanted to ask you a question."

"Yes?"

"I have an idea for using the original homestead house and the three hundred acres on the south ridge," he said.

"And?"

"And I want to talk about it. I wanted to know if you had time after dinner."

"Why not during?" Heather ventured, keeping her tone as businesslike as Reid's.

"I don't want to put you to any trouble, Miss Heather," he said slowly.

"If it were any trouble, I wouldn't have offered. Time?"

"I should be finished with my paperwork about six. Give me some time to wash and change. Seven?"

"Fine," Heather said with a nod. "Seven."

Heather turned back to the clay but did not begin to work immediately. She listened intently to Reid's fading bootfalls as he walked back along the path. When the sound of his feet were gone, she removed the towel and began to work the clay again.

Slowly, her fingers traced the nose of the bust. It was smooth, straight, and strong, with just the barest discernible notch near the ridge. Shaking her head, Heather pulled her hand away from the clay.

"Damn you!" she muttered to the sculpture. Polaris rubbed against her calf and Heather let her hand drop to his head. "I'm okay," she said to the dog as she ran her hand along the top of his head. Polaris moved again, and Heather felt him stand, placing his front paws on her shoulders. She bent, wrapping her arms around him, and nuzzled her face against his soft fur.

Heather knew that Polaris sensed her frustration, understood the need that emanated from her—the need that went unheeded by the one person who called it forth from its hidden depths.

For almost three months Reid Hunter had been the perfect foreman. Working hard, long hours, he drove himself and the men who worked for him mercilessly in an effort to reverse the decline the ranch had been in for the past two years. Never once had she heard a ranch hand complain; in fact, all she heard were murmurs of admiration and respect. Even Emma had commented on the difference of the ranch.

But Reid was an enigma to her. He was courteous to a fault, considerate of everything and everyone, and worked as hard as, if not harder than, anyone else. There were many nights that Heather heard him in the office after the ranch had quieted down for the night. Sometimes she went to him, just to talk. Other times she just listened to the low sounds of pencil on paper.

But, above it all, Reid Hunter never opened up. He never spoke about himself no matter what ploys she used. And Heather knew that tonight would be no different—that tonight she would again try to talk to him, try to get him to open up, just a little, about himself.

The table was set and everything was ready. Heather was satisfied with what she had prepared. They would start with a light onion soup, followed by sautéed chicken breasts, which she had already cooked and were being kept warm in the oven. Fresh green beans were waiting in the steamer, and when they started the soup, she would turn the burner on. Heather went to the refrigerator and checked the wine. It felt cool to the touch and she knew she'd been in time. She'd almost forgotten it. Her fingers went to her watch; he would be arriving in a few minutes.

Going to the cabinet above the sink, Heather reached up for the dishes. She took down everything she would need and then pulled out the flatware. Putting each place setting on the large plates, Heather went to the dining room table and neatly set the places. When that was done, and with a sigh, she pulled the clips from her hair and shook her head.

Feeling her hair come free, Heather smiled. She was ready. As she smoothed her dress, a simple cotton shift of soft blue, she started back toward the kitchen. When she was halfway across the floor, there was a knock on the front door.

"It's open," she called. The front door opened and closed, and she heard the now familiar pattern of Reid's boots on the floor. Before he spoke, she smelled the mild after-shave he'd used. Again Heather felt another chill of anticipation. Stop it! she admonished. But she knew it was a losing battle.

"I don't know which smells better, the food or you," Reid said in his deep voice.

"After the hours you put in today, I would imagine it's the food. Drink? Wine?"

"Sounds good," Reid commented noncommittally.

"Take a seat. I'll be right back," Heather said as she went into the kitchen.

Reid smiled at her receding back and walked over to the cordovan-covered couch. He eased himself onto the cushions and let a smile crease his face. This room was as much the essence of Heather Strand as any other part of the ranch. Reid could almost feel Heather's soft hands in the arrangement. The leather couch, so masculine, yet soft. Two matching leather chairs sat across from it, separated by a dark wooden coffee table. The paintings of landscapes and mountains decorating the off-white walls gave the living room of the Strand Ranch a homey, comfortable, and unpretentious feeling.

Reid's appraisal of the living room faded as he thought about the woman he worked for, the beauty of her face and the depth of her love for the ranch. It had been over three months since the day he had begun working for Heather, but not once in all those days had he *not* thought of the time she had told him to stop the car and of the incredible feeling of her hands as they read his face. Not one day had passed when he did not think of those hands and of the woman they were a part of.

"Do you want to give me a hint?" asked Heather as she emerged from the kitchen, a wineglass in each hand.

"A hint?"

"Thank you," Heather said with a smile. "I can't possibly know where you are if you're sitting still and not making a sound."

"Oh? I would have thought you could hear me breathing, with your hearing."

"It's not quite that good, but I'm trying," Heather said. Reid stood and took one of the wineglasses.

Heather nodded to him, walked to the couch, and sat down. Reid sat on the opposite end and waited.

"Well?" Heather asked.

"Well, what?"

"You said you wanted to talk with me," she reminded him. Reid looked at her, unable to take his eyes from her face. She wore very little makeup, just a bit of lipstick and some blue eyeshadow. He almost asked her how she put it on, but stopped himself just in time.

"You look very pretty tonight. Blue suits you."

"Thank you," Heather said, enjoying the warmth his words gave her. "And?"

"And I have an idea, but it will take a while to put it all together. We won't be able to start utilizing it until next summer," Reid began. Heather sensed a strange hesitation in his voice, one she had never heard before in their short acquaintance. The hesitation made her wonder exactly what Reid was trying to lead into.

Heather sipped the cooled wine. Placing the glass on the coffee table, she sat further back on the couch, lifted her legs, and tucked them under her. Then, as she smoothed her dress over her folded legs, she spoke. "Will it cost a lot of money?"

"A bit," he replied.

"Then I guess we can forget it. The banks won't loan us any more money until we can show them an upswing on sales."

"I have another source for the loan," Reid informed her.

"I thought loan sharks operated out of big cities," Heather joked.

"It's not a loan shark," Reid said, ignoring Heather's attempt at humor. "It's a foundation." Heather heard Reid take a deep breath and prepared herself for something different.

Reid glanced from Heather to his wineglass and back again. He knew it would be hard for a rancher, man or woman, to separate from their property, to utilize it for something out of the ordinary. But what he had in mind would be beneficial to both the ranch and the people it involved.

"There is a charitable organization that grants loans to businesses in exchange for the use of some of their facilities or for the use of some of their employees. I have a contact in that organization, and my idea would help both the ranch and them."

"You mean, if I were to lease some of the Strand land to them or hire some of their people, I could get the money we need?" Heather asked. She knew the surprise she felt was evident in her voice, but this was too important to try to hide it.

"It's a little more involved than that," Reid started.

Heather interrupted him with a raised hand. "In that case, I think we should eat," she said as she stood. Reid stood also and walked over to her. He took her elbow and guided her into the dining room. Heather did not fight his touch, and only when they were in the dining room did she pull away.

"Please sit," she said as she pointed unerringly to one of the place settings. "I'll get the soup." Inside the kitchen, Heather poured the steaming liquid into two white china bowls. She paused for a moment as she felt her hands shake. *Relax!* she ordered herself. *He's just your foreman. Nothing else!*

Polaris's low whine called to her. She turned to the dog and patted her shoulders. Polaris jumped up and nuzzled her cheek. "You're a good boy," she said as she straightened up and let Polaris go. "Run!" she ordered.

Polaris barked once, but did not leave. "Go ahead, boy," she said. She heard Polaris walk to the door that separated the kitchen from the dining room and whine. Heather smiled, touched by the dog's loyalty when there was another in the house. "Run!" she repeated the order. Polaris barked and finally left through his special door. "I wish I had a good enough reason to need you near me," she whispered to the now absent dog.

Reid watched Heather pour the coffee as he sat back, filled and contented from the wonderfully prepared meal. As if by mutual consent, neither of them had spoken of the loan or the use of the three hundred acres. But now, with dinner over, and even though he wanted to postpone the inevitable, Reid began to speak. Before he could say more than three words, Heather interrupted him.

"Wait until we've finished our coffee. I have a feeling that I want to enjoy the peace for a few more minutes."

Reid laughed at her words and agreed. "Miss Heather," Reid said.

"Heather! I won't tell you again—after hours you call me Heather," she ordered with a bantering scowl.

"Yes, ma'am," Reid drawled, liking the crease that furrowed her brow. As he spoke, Heather's face relaxed. "Heather, for the last month everyone's been wondering what you're working on. The boys tell me that you always let everyone watch you work. But for the last month . . ." Heather knew the question was destined to be asked, but somehow she had hoped to avoid it.

"Sometimes an artist needs privacy to work. I need it right now," she said. Heather didn't like the way her voice sounded. The lie didn't ring right and she was afraid that Reid would pick up on it. "Are you finished with your coffee?" she asked suddenly.

"Yes, ma'am," Reid replied.

"Take me for a walk and tell me about your idea," she said. Heather sat still as she listened to Reid's chair brush along the carpet. She knew when he stepped behind her chair and stood just as he pulled the chair out for her. Then his hand was on her elbow. His hands, calloused and hard, felt good on her skin, comfortable and exciting at the same time. The gentle warmth of his palm, as it cupped her elbow, threatened to turn her legs to rubber. She stayed silent, content to be guided out of the house. Heather paused momentarily to lift her shawl free from the rack.

The night air was cool, as most June nights were in

the mountains, and Heather breathed deeply, taking in all the scents of the ranch. The horses, the flowers, and the freshly baled hay seemed to send out messages of peace to her. The tall man who walked next to her, his hand never leaving her arm, gave her comfort.

Heather was so involved in her thoughts that she almost missed Reid's first words. Pulling her mind from its random wandering, Heather listened intently.

"My idea is to lease the three hundred acres to the New Life Foundation, to use the land and the house for a summer camp for teens, and to hire eligible men and women who need jobs and train them as counselors and ranch hands. The camp would be set up as a miniature working ranch. The campers would be the actual ranch hands. They would learn to ride and to handle the real chores of a ranch."

"That's marvelous," Heather said, liking the idea instantly. "But why would this foundation be willing to give us money to keep the ranch going when they could just as easily buy another ranch and convert the entire property into a camp?"

"They don't want to be involved in the year-round running of a ranch. Something like this gives them the opportunity to have knowledgeable, skilled people on hand if problems develop. Besides, the camp is only run for three months. The expenses to keep it operating year-round would be exorbitant," Reid added.

"From the sound of your voice, I think you've already spoken to some people about this," Heather ventured.

"Yes, ma'am," Reid replied, and Heather caught the humor in his words.

"I'll have to think about it," she told him. "Reid, how much money do you think we really need to get this ranch back on its feet?"

Reid looked at her in the soft moonlight. He felt his blood race as his eyes traced the shadows on her face. He knew he was on dangerous ground emotionally. Before he answered, he forced away the feelings of need that kept surfacing when she was near.

"We're doing okay right now, but the sales of the horses are slow and prices have been pushed down. I have a feeling that if you hold out for another six months things will get better."

"You haven't answered my question."

"About fifty thousand dollars," he said bluntly.

"But . . . ." Heather began, stunned at the magnitude of the amount. "I thought we were doing better. . . . I thought you had things turning around."

"I do. But your old foreman sold off the two best breeders when he tried to raise the money to keep things going. We need another good stud, maybe two. That and enough money to keep the boys happy," Reid finished.

"Hank said we had enough good breeders," Heather said, defending the old foreman pointlessly. Her mind was numbed from the shock of Reid's assessment; she had been betrayed by Hank Thompson, betrayed and hurt.

"I'm sure he thought you did, but he was wrong. Heather, what's been done in the past can't be changed. I've checked on a lot of things, and what I found was that your father was the real foreman here. Thompson only carried out his orders. The man never made a decision on his own. He was too afraid of the consequences. Your father knew that, but also appreciated Thompson's strong points. That was why he kept him on. Now, my job, and yours, is very simple. We must rebuild the ranch. We're on our way, and the foundation will lend you the money at a low interest rate. My advice, as your foreman and general manager, is to take the loan."

"Thank you, Reid," Heather said as she turned to face him. She could feel the heat of his body reach out to her. She longed to be held in his strong arms. Without realizing it, Heather raised one hand to Reid's face. She traced his jawline, feeling again the strength under the skin. Her fingers lingered for a moment before she withdrew her hand.

"Thank you," she repeated. Turning from him, Heather began her lonely walk back to the house.

As she neared the front steps, Reid saw Polaris emerge from the night to walk beside his mistress. He stood there, silently watching, as Heather disappeared into the house.

Reid had decided during dinner that he would not hide the ranch's financial condition from Heather. Everyone had been doing that for the last year, trying to protect her from the knowledge that the Strand Ranch was almost bankrupt. Tom, with his past banking experience, Emma, and even a few of the regular ranch hands knew what was happening. Each had contributed whatever they could to keep the ranch alive. But tonight he knew if he was going to help her and the ranch, he had to make Heather aware of the true situation.

The New Life Foundation was a small organization, relatively unknown, and one that maintained a low profile. It was an organization that helped both the surviving veterans of the Vietnam War and the children of the refugees who were driven from their homeland. Reid knew the foundation would loan the Strand Ranch the money it needed in exchange for the use of the land and the training that the ranch's cowboys would give their own employees. It would be a good business decision for Heather Strand and the right move for the people who needed the ranch property.

Reid continued to watch the main house, leaning against the corral fence until he saw each light in the house extinguished. Then he smiled as he walked back to his own quarters. Heather had no need for light at night, and he'd once asked her why she used them.

"It makes the other people on the ranch feel good to see lights on in the main house," she'd told him simply. She was quite a lady, Reid Hunter thought.

Chapter Six

Heather could hear everything. Every sound the house made was usually an old friend to her. But tonight, as she tried to sleep, her old friends seemed to be conspiring against her. The breeze that came through the opened living room window pushed the drapes against the windowframe, and even though it hardly made a sound, in Heather's ears it was loud.

Each time she shifted on the large bed, searching for a comfortable position, she became even more restless. With a sigh, Heather sat up and leaned against the headboard. Reaching onto the night table, Heather felt for the book that was there. With another sigh she opened the book at her place mark and began to read. The raised characters of the braille alphabet were soothing against the sensitive tips of her fingers, but the words she read seemed disjointed and meaningless.

Slamming the book closed, Heather shook her head.

She knew what was wrong, but she did not know what she could do about it. He was so . . . so much a cowboy! she thought angrily.

Heather reached for her watch and read the time. Although it was one in the morning, she left the bed and slipped on a pair of jeans and a flannel shirt. Then, after putting on her boots, she called Polaris.

"Stay," she commanded him as she left the house.

After Heather had left Reid, she'd thought about what he'd said. She knew he'd been speaking the truth about the state of the ranch and also knew that unless something happened soon she would lose it. Heather almost laughed, remembering the cartoons she'd listened to when she was a child, about the bad men who tried to steal the ranch from the helpless heroine.

Only this was real, and she could do something about it. She and Reid. Slowly, as Heather walked from the main house, she made her decision.

Heather knew every inch of this part of the ranch as well as she knew her studio. But she was surprised when she found herself, unplanned, at the steps that led to Reid's front door.

As on most ranches, the foreman and several of the men who lived with their families had small houses. The rest of the men lived in the traditional bunkhouses. Now, after climbing the steps to the porch and standing at Reid's door, Heather hesitated for a moment.

Should she wake him, she wondered, and tell him she'd made her decision? Or was the truth that she had made the decision now so that she could talk to him again tonight?

Taking a deep breath, Heather raised her hand to knock.

"No one's home," came the deep voice of Heather's foreman. She turned quickly in the direction the voice had issued from. There was a small porch, with two chairs on it. Heather knew that Reid was sitting in one of them.

Her heart pounded as she started to walk toward him. "I thought you'd be sleeping," she said.

"I was, for a while," he admitted.

"I couldn't sleep either," she said, then let out a self-conscious laugh. "But I guess that's evident."

"I guess."

Heather felt Reid grasp her hand and hold it until she sat. She didn't trust her voice yet and was quiet as his hand left hers. "Your tobacco smells nice," she said as she sniffed the fragrance of the smoke he had just lit.

Silence greeted her words. Heather knew that she must do something, say something about why she was here. "Reid . . ."

"It's okay, Heather. When you can't sleep, having company is nice. You don't have to make excuses."

"I'm not," she began, knowing she was. "Will you hold my hand?" she asked in a low voice. Even as the words left her lips, she felt her heart race and her breathing deepen. Then the hard warmth of his hand enfolded hers.

"I lied before," she said suddenly, but noticed that the pressure of his hand on hers did not change as she spoke. "About when you asked what I was working on in the studio. I'm doing a sculpture of you."

"Why?"

"Because I want to. Reid, I've made my decision," she said. Again there was only silence and the heat from his hand. "You can make the arrangements for the loan and draw up the lease for the land and the homestead, on one condition." Heather paused again, but could detect nothing, not even a change in breathing from Reid. "Are you still awake?"

"No man alive could fall asleep holding your hand," he said. Heather's breath was tight in her throat as she forced herself to speak.

"The condition is simple—I can't finish the bust without you. I want you to model for me." Once the words were out, Heather felt both relieved and yet even more nervous. She hadn't planned on adding the condition, but now that she had, she was glad.

"Heather," Reid began hesitantly, "I don't think . . . I mean, I can't take time off during the day."

"I know. We'll do it at night. It won't take long," she told him. "Only a few sessions."

"I . . . all right," he said. Then he stood, pulling her to her feet. "Let me walk with you back to the house."

Heather didn't argue as he led her down the steps and across the flat ground toward her house. She had not let go of his hand and could feel the muscles within it. From the moment he'd first touched her hand, heat had spread upward along her arm. Now the heat filled her entire body. It was strange, but what was most frightening was the knowledge that just holding his hand was not enough. It would never be enough.

Suddenly they were at her door. She turned to face him, and without willing it, she pulled her hand from his and lifted it to his face. Her other hand rose also and went to his shoulder. She felt his body become tense as her hand slipped to the back of his neck. She felt the muscles that knotted in warning, but could not stop herself or what was happening. She pulled his head down and felt his resistance leave. As their mouths met, hers exploded with the sensation of his lips pressing against hers. His arms were suddenly around her, crushing her to his chest.

Heather couldn't breathe as tiny lances of fire shot through her body. Her breasts, flattened against him, seemed to swell, and his hands, in the small of her back, were like twin brands. The taste of his mouth on hers, the slight scent of tobacco on his mustache, and the power and strength of his body against hers drove all thoughts from her mind. The only thing Heather was conscious of was an overwhelming desire to be part of Reid Hunter.

Then Reid pulled his lips from hers and she heard the harsh exhalation that came from his mouth. It matched hers in both intensity and need. They clung together like castaways in an ocean with only each other to help themselves stay afloat. Above the hammering of her heart, Heather heard Reid's whisper.

"We can't," Reid said, as he forced himself to regain control of his mind and body. The softness that was pressed so closely to him made his head swim and his body ache. "That was wrong of me. I'm sorry," he said, pulling away gently.

Heather tried to force her breathing back to normal as she held her balled fists against her sides. She did not try to hide how she felt about him, but would not allow him to see the effects of his rejection. She had been stupidly foolish to let her emotions take charge of her actions.

"You have nothing to be sorry about," Heather informed him in as cool a voice as she could muster.

"I have a lot to be sorry about. One of those things is that I work for you. If I didn't, things could be different. But I am working for you, and what just happened should not have."

"Reid, it won't make any difference to the men," she told him.

"Yes, it will. We don't live in a big city where no one cares about who does what to whom. We live in a closed environment where everyone knows everyone else's business. The hands won't work for the owner of a ranch who comes down to them."

"You're wrong! This is not eighteen-eighty Nevada. This is today!" Heather argued, already knowing the futility of it.

"More so even now. The men work for you and respect you. But if push came to shove and they found out that you were playing with the help, they'd all leave," Reid stated.

"I don't think so," she said in challenge. Her mind reeled from his words, but she would not let herself accept them. "Is it really because I'm the boss, or is it because I'm blind?" Heather asked in an unthinking whisper.

"You can probably see more with your hands and ears than someone else does with their eyes. No, Heather—you're the boss, I'm the hired help. And that's the way it has to be."

Heather refused to listen to any more. She didn't want to believe him about the hired-hand relationship, but she knew that what Reid had described could happen. It wouldn't be the first time. She had heard stories about women ranchers and what had happened to them.

"All right, then I too have to say I'm sorry."

"Good night, Heather," Reid said in a low, gentle voice.

"Good night, Reid," she replied, holding back the sob that was trying to force itself past her lips. She turned and went up the steps and into the welcome security of her house. Once inside, she ran into her bedroom and collapsed on the bed.

"I will not cry!" she told herself in a husky voice, "I will not!" Then she felt the warmth and softness of

Polaris as he pressed his muzzle into her side. Heather sat up, pulling the dog's large head onto her lap. She stroked the domed head for a few minutes until she had all her emotions under control.

"Damn you, Reid Hunter! I'm not finished with you and your archaic rules!"

Chapter Seven

Heather awoke to the sounds of the ranch coming to life. Every day, except for Sunday, was the same. The early-morning sounds of the men going to breakfast were followed by the men getting their horses and riding out to assignments Reid had given them. She could tell to the minute what time it was by what the men were doing.

Listening to the first pair of riders leaving the corral, Heather knew it was six o'clock. She had slept later than usual, and the first things she had been aware of were the ranch hands. Now, as she listened to the riders, her memory of the previous night returned with a painful rush.

How could she have done what she did? How could she have let her emotions rule her as they had last night? Could she even talk to Reid today? But, what was worse, Heather thought as she threw the blanket from her, was that she wanted to be kissed and held within Reid's strong arms. She wanted to be with him as she had never before wanted anything.

Then another memory returned—the kiss that she and Reid had shared and her instant reaction to it. Even as she thought about it, she could feel her body reacting again as it had the night before. Her stomach fluttered and her breathing grew ragged. Her legs felt weak and her breasts became sensitive and tender. "Stop it!" she ordered in a loud voice. Suddenly Polaris jumped up and barked.

"Not you," she said as she scratched behind his ear and laughed. "Me," she added. Grateful for the dog's ability to break her mood, Heather rose and dressed. She, too, had a full schedule today and wanted an early start. After breakfast she had work to do in the studio. After that, she was going into town with Emma to get supplies for her studio and to teach her weekly art class at the senior citizens' center.

As Heather emerged from the bedroom, she smelled bacon cooking and went into the kitchen. "My you're up late today," said Emma Kline. "Hot date?" she kidded.

"Couldn't get to sleep. You're in early," Heather said with a smile, forcing herself to play the part.

"Lots of work to be done if I'm chauffeuring you about today. Anyway, sleepyhead, I thought you might like some breakfast. You've got a long day ahead of you, too."

"Thank you," Heather said as she moved to the sink and reached for the percolator.

"Already made," Emma informed her. "Don't you dare!" she ordered as Heather began to make a face. "My coffee's just as good as yours—better, as a matter of fact!"

"If you like mud," Heather retorted, but smiled as she did.

"Humph," was Emma's only reply. "Sit," she said, and Heather went to the table. Heather suddenly realized she was hungry and ate as soon as the food was placed before her.

"Emma?" Heather called as she put her fork down on the empty plate.

"Still hungry?"

"No. Why didn't you tell me how bad off the ranch really was?"

"Who said it was so bad?"

"Reid."

"That's why you couldn't sleep, wasn't it?" asked the woman who had become her closest friend.

"Partially. Emma, how long were you going to keep it from me?"

"Listen, hon, Tom and I talked it out, and we thought we had a pretty good chance of keeping the ranch going. When you hired Reid Hunter, we knew we had a foreman who could keep us going. Now I'm not so sure," Emma finished.

"I really appreciate what you've done, but I do wish you had told me. Maybe I could have done something to help in the beginning."

"Not after what Hank Thompson did. Only a miracle could have helped."

"So Reid said."

"What else did he say?" Emma asked in a guarded tone.

"Stop that!" Heather told her crisply. "He said we need about fifty thousand dollars to get back on our feet."

"That's about right," admitted the bookkeeper.

"Reid is getting us a loan." Heather thought Emma would say something, but all she heard was absolute silence. "Emma?"

"What do you have to give up for it?" Emma asked in a strangely subdued voice.

"What do you mean?"

"Money is tight. Tighter than I've ever seen it. How can an itinerant cowboy get you a fifty-thousand-dollar loan? You have to give up something for it. What?"

"Emma, I thought you liked Reid," she said, hiding the smile that tried to escape.

"I do. But as old as I am, I've learned a lot. You just don't get something for nothing."

"Okay, you're right," Heather said. Then, for effect, she lowered her voice, putting sadness into it. "I'm giving up the south ridge three hundred for—"

"The old homestead?" Emma interrupted, her voice hushed and far away. "Your father's turning over in his grave."

"A camp," she finished. It took Emma a few seconds for the last words to register, and Heather finally allowed the smile to reach her lips.

"A camp?" came the questioning echo.

"The loan is from a foundation. It's a low-interest note," she told the bookkeeper, and then explained the entire situation. When she was finished, Heather knew there was a smile spread across Emma's face. And she knew she had made the right decision.

Heather stood alone in the studio, waiting. It had been two nights since she had spoken to Reid about sitting for the sculpture, and tonight was to be their first session. She was nervous, almost afraid, of his arrival. For the last two days, it had been relatively easy. There were always people around, and both she and Reid had acted normally. But tonight they would be alone again.

Heather went to the clay and let her fingers roam over the surface of the partially completed sculpture. The nose was almost finished and the eyes had been outlined well. She wanted to recheck them, not trusting her memory of one time to be as accurate as she wanted.

Again Heather thought about that night and the kiss they had shared and the words that had been spoken. Since she had been a child, she had always gone after what she wanted—more so because she was blind. Heather had built her inner strength to a point that refused to allow her to give up on any goal she had set for herself. This part of her demanded she fight for it—perhaps, she thought, because she was blind and had to rely on herself and her instincts more than she would have had to had she had her sight. And Heather knew she wanted Reid Hunter. But she also wanted more than just an affair.

She was so absorbed in her thoughts, she did not hear Reid enter the studio.

"Miss Heather?" she heard him call.

"I thought we agreed about that," she said.

"We did. But . . ." Reid left the rest unsaid.

"All right, Reid, we'll play by your antiquated rules. I guess I don't have much choice. Sit over here," she told him, pointing to the same stool he had first seen Gregg on.

Reid watched her face as she spoke, feeling each word she said as if they were being shot at him. He shook his head, sad to be hurting her but knowing it was for the best. Even as he moved and watched her moisten the clay, he felt his desire stir again. With the iron willpower of years of practice, Reid forced the emotion down and made himself comfortable on the stool.

"I'm ready," he said.

"Yes, sir," she replied.

Feeling her heart begin its increased pounding, Heather walked to him. When her thigh touched his knee, she paused. Then, slowly, she raised her hands and began to "see" his face.

She started with his eyes, gently passing her fingers across them, feeling the softness of the lids and the feathery fineness of his eyelashes. Her fingers glided over his eyebrows and then along the sides of his eyes. She felt the indented lines of the crows-feet, and her stomach fluttered again.

"Smile." He did, and the lines beneath her fingers furrowed deeper, and she explored these to their ends. Slowly, reluctantly, she drew her hands away. "You can relax for a few minutes," she told him as she walked back to the clay.

There she began to work on the eyes. As she did, she sensed Reid behind her, studying the work she had already done. "It's still in the roughest stage."

"How long have you been working on it?" he asked.

"Almost a month," she answered honestly.

"I think the nose is a touch big."

"No, it's exact."

"You only *saw* it once."

"It *made* an impression. Be quiet for a few minutes and let me work."

"Yes, ma'am."

"And stop calling me ma'am!" she yelled, louder than she'd intended. "Sorry."

Reid didn't reply as he backed away from her. He

knew he shouldn't push that hard, but he was trying to lighten things up. He returned to the stool, contenting himself with watching her work.

"Reid?" Heather called softly as her fingers molded the clay.

"Yes."

"Do you always stay up that late?"

"I wasn't up," Reid said, knowing what she was talking about and surprised that he was admitting the truth. "I woke up and couldn't go back to sleep."

"Does it happen a lot?"

"Enough," he replied. Heather sensed intuitively that something was hidden behind his words but decided not to force it.

For the next fifteen minutes Heather's fingers probed, patted, and smoothed the clay until she had what she wanted. When she was satisfied, she dipped her hands in the basin, rinsing off the clay, and then dried them.

"The forehead now," she said as she moved to Reid again. Her hands went to his skin, and she traced the area from his eyebrows to his hairline. She followed the hairline until it ended in sideburns and then returned to his forehead. She traced the three deep grooves that were there, and then made him wrinkle his forehead to better grasp the mobility of his face. When she was done, she left him quickly and returned to the clay.

It had been easier this time, Heather realized. She had her emotions under control and refused to allow her body to betray her. If he didn't want her, she would not force herself on him. At least, that's what she tried to tell herself, until she remembered the intensity of his kiss and the way he had drawn her to him. He wanted her and she knew it.

"Do you dream a lot?" Heather asked, using her words to break the patterns her thoughts were taking.

"A fair amount."

"What's it like?" she asked.

"My dreams?" Reid's voice sounded strained to Heather's ears.

"I'm not trying to pry into your dreams. Just to make conversation," she said. "I dream, but mine are very different. I've been told about dreaming in color, about seeing things that are both real and surreal. I was just wondering about yours."

"Why are yours different?" Reid asked. The moment the words left his mouth he'd realized how foolish they were. "That was a stupid question," he said.

"Not really," Heather told him. "You have to understand that I've never seen, ever, and I don't know what color is like. In my dreams I can hear, feel, and I guess see, but I'm not sure. I think when I see in my dreams that what I'm seeing is my imagination."

"I'd trade imagination for reality," Reid said suddenly.

Heather felt a different type of tension fill the air after Reid had spoken. Before there had been an electricity that had permeated the studio, making them careful. Now the charged atmosphere seemed directed toward Reid and his words.

"Is that why you haven't settled down yet?" Heather asked, holding her breath as she did.

"Partly," said Reid. "How's the sculpture coming?" he asked, changing the subject and his voice at the same time. He was getting into dangerous water and he didn't want to pursue it any further.

"I'll respect your privacy, Mr. Hunter."

"Thank you."

"You're welcome," Heather said quickly. Then she began to laugh. When she had herself settled down, she finally spoke. "You know, Mr. Hunter, we're both adults who are in a . . . a different situation. Why don't we try to relax and enjoy each other's company instead of being so formal?"

"Miss Heather . . ."

"Can't you understand? Reid, I'm trying to be friendly. I'm trying to pretend the other night never happened. I'm trying to make you relax."

Reid looked at her for a long-drawn-out moment before he spoke. "I know. And I appreciate it, Heather."

"Good. Now, I'm finished with you for tonight. You're free to go."

"I don't think so," he murmured in a barely audible whisper. Heather caught herself and did not let him know she had heard. Even as low as the words were, they sent a thrill racing through her. "I'll see you in the morning," Reid said.

"Good night," Heather replied as she turned back to the clay.

Reid left then, walking slowly, taking his time. His thoughts were focused on Heather Strand, and nothing seemed to be able to tear them away. Reid knew he should leave, get his things together and get the hell away. He was playing with fire, and although he didn't care if he was burned, he didn't want her hurt. And he knew that if he became involved with her she would be hurt. Heather had suffered enough in her life without adding Reid's problems to it.

Reid stopped on the porch of his small house and sat on one of the chairs. He lit a cigarillo, drawing deeply on the smoke as he tried to force away, again, the emotions that kept filling his thoughts.

Chapter Eight

*E*ach evening meal was getting harder to finish, knowing that afterward she would go to the studio, meet Reid, work on the sculpture, and "see" his face. Heather was almost finished with him, as far as needing him to sit. All the rough sculpting was completed except for a few minor details which would be taken care of tonight, she thought as her blood pounded in her ears.

No, the hard part was acting normal, pretending that she felt nothing for him and knowing deep down within her that he felt the same attraction toward her.

Heather admitted she was confused, to herself at least, about why she felt the way she did toward Reid. She didn't want to. She didn't want any emotional entanglement in her life. She had sworn after that one time in college that she would not have a man in her life. She had her art and the ranch, and that was all she needed. But her dreams and her thoughts all called her a liar.

The sound of the typewriter in the office reminded her that Emma was still hard at work. Emma needed to be off tomorrow, Friday, and in order to do so she had to set up the payroll today for Reid to have on Saturday.

Heather took her plate with the half-eaten food on it to the sink. She put it down and turned. She needed to talk to someone, and the only woman she could speak with was Emma.

She walked through the house quietly, trying to build up enough courage to tell her friend her problem and at the same time to be open and honest about it. That was the problem—the honesty. Reid had put enough doubt into her mind, when he'd told her why they could not be lovers to make her wonder about seeking Emma's counsel. As she opened the office door, Heather began to doubt the wisdom of what she was doing.

The typewriter stopped its clacking as soon as Heather stepped inside. "Hi, hon. Finished with dinner?"

"Yes. I just stopped by to see how you're doing," Heather said.

"Another hour and I'll be finished."

"Excited?" Heather asked.

"At my age, if I got too excited I'd have a heart attack," Emma informed her gravely.

"Stop being so blasé. You haven't seen your nephew in five years. You have to be excited."

"I am, hon, believe me I am. You know, he graduated with honors and he's been accepted for his residency at Johns Hopkins. We finally have someone with brains in the family," Emma finished proudly.

"Besides you, you mean," Heather added. But she

knew the smile she put on her mouth didn't look as happy as she sounded.

"How's your latest model doing?"

"Fine," she replied, fighting the quaver in her voice.

"Look, young lady, I've been watching you mope around here for days. What's wrong?"

"Nothing."

"You don't look like nothing."

"I don't know how I look," she snapped back.

"But you know how you sound. C'mon, hon, this is Emma you're talking to. 'Fess up," she admonished, undaunted by Heather's sharp words.

"You know, I came in here to talk to you but I don't think I'm ready yet," Heather said truthfully.

"Well, then, as down at the mouth as you look, I guess I'll just have to cancel my trip. I don't want to be a thousand miles away thinking that you might need me."

"You'll do nothing of the sort! You're going to visit your family, and that's all there is to it!" Heather heard Emma shift in the chair and heard that funny sound that she always associated with Emma, a soft whooshing of the chair seat filling with air as Emma stood. Heather knew she was standing now. She regretted her decision to speak to Emma and should have realized that she had to work it out by herself.

"Really, Emma, it's something I have to handle myself."

"You know what? I think you can't handle this yourself. You never come to me when you should. What is it? Is it a man?"

Heather wondered if Emma could read her mind. It wasn't the first time she'd thought that, either. She nodded her head slightly.

"Do I know him?" Emma probed. This time Heather shook her head. "Heather," Emma began, and Heather felt her friend's arm fall comfortingly around her shoulders. "I know everything that happens at this ranch. And I know there hasn't been any man a-callin' on you."

"It's someone on the ranch, and that's the problem," Heather admitted in a hushed voice, secure in Emma's warmth.

"He's a hell of a man," Emma said.

"You don't know who it is."

"Heather, since the day Reid Hunter started here, I've seen the change in you. It was only a matter of time before you admitted it."

"But it doesn't make any difference. I'm the boss and he's the foreman. Besides, who'd want a blind woman?" Heather finished bitterly.

She felt Emma stiffen next to her and then relax. "I've never heard you say anything so foolish in all the time I've known you."

"Well, I feel foolish."

"But you're not an idiot. Being blind has nothing to do with it."

"I know," Heather whispered, "but it's either that, or I'm not pretty enough, or . . ." Emma interrupted her before she could think of anything else.

"He's too damned young to be one of the old breed. But he is, isn't he?" Emma asked.

"Yes."

"Do you really feel it, deep down in your heart?" Emma asked in a hushed voice. Heather nodded slowly. "How does he feel?"

"I . . . I don't know. I think he feels the same way, but all he said to me was that it can't be."

"I know the feeling. Heather, I'm going to give you

some advice. You can take him or leave him, that's up to you. But if you don't take him, you'll have only yourself to blame."

Heather heard what her friend said, but only the first words really penetrated. "You know the feeling?" she echoed.

Emma's voice sounded far away and sad as she spoke. "Yes, I know the feeling. What you're going through happened to me thirty years ago."

Emma sighed, then guided Heather to a chair next to hers. When both women were seated, Emma started speaking again.

"I was almost twenty. My father owned a small ranch outside of Butte. We had fifteen hands working for us, and one of them—Jim Garber was his name—was the most handsome, devil-may-care cowboy you ever met. The minute I saw him, I fell in love. He was tall, and slim, and sat in a saddle like he was born to it.

"Well, it was during the summer that I started riding in the evenings—just a little ride while there was still light. I would ride out from the ranch—not far—and enjoy the land and the early stars that were beginning to come out. After about a week, I had company. Jim started to ride with me. He'd meet me after I was already riding, and we'd ride for half an hour, never speaking, just riding and enjoying the horses and the country.

"I don't know how it started, but one night we ended up in each other's arms. Heather, it was beautiful. I was in love, and he was in love with me. Well, that night, as we returned to the house, Jim stopped where he always did and said good night. I didn't understand. We were in love, and there was nothing wrong with it.

"That was when I learned the rules. He got off his horse and helped me down. We walked, and he talked.

He told me why no one could ever know about what had happened. He told me that if we wanted to keep on seeing each other it would have to be that way. I argued with him, told him my father wouldn't care.

"He said to me that even if my father didn't mind, the rest of the boys would. They would think he was trying to marry into the ranch. I told him we'd run away. He said no. It wouldn't work that way.

"No matter how much I cried, no matter what I said, I couldn't shake the way he felt. I learned a lot that night, and over the next weeks I found out more. I talked with my friends and listened to what they said. Jim had been right. It would never work."

"So you didn't see him anymore?" Heather asked, almost biting her lip at her interruption.

"It wasn't that easy. I told you I was in love with him. I was, deeply, and he was in love with me. We kept on seeing each other for almost two years, living a secret life that was hell. I wouldn't give him up, and he wouldn't bend an inch. Finally, the day came that he told me he was leaving, that he had to leave so that I could find someone else and have a real life.

"I begged him not to go, that there was no one else for me. A week later Jim was gone. I never saw him again. And I never found anyone I could love as much again." When Emma finished, Heather raised her hands to her friend's face. She felt the tears on Emma's cheeks and pulled her friend into her arms. After a few moments Emma drew away.

"Now, I told you that story for only one reason. To make you to see what you might be getting yourself into and to see that Reid was telling you the truth, as far as he can see it."

"Did you regret it?" Heather asked.

Emma took her hand and squeezed it gently. "Not

for one minute. I had two years with the man I love, and it's lasted me a lifetime. I wouldn't have given that up for anything."

"Then you think I should . . ."

"I don't think anything," Emma interrupted. "My advice is simple. Do what you have to, but if you decide to force things with Reid, go in with your mind open and know what the end results might be. But I have to tell you something else. Reid Hunter is no ordinary ranch hand. I don't know why I feel that, but I do. There's more to him than just being a cowboy."

"I know. Emma, thank you. Don't worry about me. Enjoy your family."

"I will. And, Heather, you're my family also. Don't forget that either."

"I won't," Heather said as she stood and started to the door. She touched the dial of her watch and knew Reid would be waiting. "I'll see you on Monday," she said as she closed the office door.

Heather stood in the studio, her hands clean from the clay, and finished for the night. The session had gone smoothly and Heather knew she had been unusually quiet. Emma's words kept echoing in her mind as she worked, and she would not trust her voice to keep up any real conversation. She knew that Reid had noticed her silence, but he had been good enough not to say anything. Now, she thought, she should go to bed and sleep, but she knew that tonight, like that night weeks ago, she would find sleep a hard sanctuary to find.

Heather closed the studio and walked toward the corral. She had no destination in mind, but had a need for physical activity. She walked slowly, with even strides, Polaris at her side. The evening air was warm—unusually warm and still for this time of year. Next month it would get warmer, but nothing like the lowlands. She was glad she wore only a light cotton top and her jeans.

The sounds of the night whispered to her as she reached the corral. Instead of stopping, Heather turned and walked to the far side, toward the large pond, two hundred yards past the corral. This was the pond where her father had taught her to swim, and it was a place where she had spent many summer days sitting, letting her legs soak in the water as she played.

As these memories welled up in her mind, she thought about her father and mother. Then she thought about her father and what his reaction would be to Reid Hunter. Would he have been against her and Reid? No, she had known her father well enough to believe that he would have smiled on his daughter's love.

Suddenly Polaris blocked her way and Heather knew she was at the pond's edge. "Good boy," she said as she ruffled the fur on his head and sat down. Bending, she dipped her fingers into the pond's pleasantly cool water. Then she removed her boots and rolled up her jeans to let her feet feel the coolness.

Reid and Tom Farley sat in Tom's kitchen, talking about one of the problems that had cropped up during the day. They had spent the last two hours trying to iron it out. After the second cup of coffee for Reid and the third for Tom, they decided to try out their idea. Reid smiled as he stood and offered his hand. Tom Farley took it with a matching smile.

"I really appreciate the way you've been helping me out," Reid said as he withdrew his hand.

"I knew the shape the ranch was in better than anyone. I'm sure glad you came along when you did. I think Heather feels the same way."

"Thanks, Tom," Reid said with a nod. Then his assistant walked him to the door and bid him good night. Outside, Reid paused as he looked up at the stars. It was a clear night, cloudless, with a small crescent moon riding low in the sky. The warm air smelled clean, and the ranch was quiet. Reid began to walk toward his house, but felt restless with excess energy.

He had hoped, when he saw Tom's kitchen light on, that talking with the man would take some of the edge from him. He'd been wrong. Reid knew it was more than just unused energy that was coarsing through his body. Tonight, sitting for Heather, watching her work on the sculpture of his face, had been the hardest part of his day. He knew it had been the last night he would be sitting, and although he was glad, he was also sorry that he would not be able to spend more evenings alone with her, even if all he could do was watch her.

Walking along the path that led to his house, Reid saw, out of the corner of his eye, a shadow walk by the corral. He stopped, prepared for anything, but most especially a mountain cat. He turned slowly, breathing a sigh of relief. He saw two shapes and knew it was Heather because of the four-legged silhouette trotting next to her.

Reid stayed still and watched her walk toward the pond. Suddenly he felt a warning chill but fought it off. She had lived here all her life and knew every part of this ranch. If she was going to the pond, it was because she wanted to.

But even though the logic was sound, Reid did not want to think of what might happen if she accidentally stumbled into the water. He waited a few more minutes after Heather had been swallowed by the darkness before he began to follow her.

When he was twenty yards from the pond, he saw her silhouette. She was standing sideways to him, knee deep in the water, Polaris at her side. His breath caught in his throat. She had shed her clothing, and the moonlight shaded her skin as if she were a painting. Reid knew he should leave, should take his eyes from her, but he could not. Her body was too perfect, the smooth-flowing lines all cried out to him. Her high breasts stood proudly, a graceful arc in the night. Her stomach was flat, and her back curved delicately inward, blending into a tight, well-molded derrière that made his blood run fast.

He was rooted to the spot, captured by her lonely beauty, but he knew he could not move forward, could not reveal himself. Reid stood like a statue and waited until Heather dipped down into the water and began to swim. His desire fled as a new worry crept into his mind. She was blind. She couldn't know where she was swimming to. Suddenly he saw the wake created by Polaris's head near hers, guiding her around in the water.

Reid shook his head in wonder of the capabilities of the dog. A few minutes later, Heather and the dog came out of the pond at the exact spot where a dark pile of clothing waited.

As Heather lay down on the grass, Reid breathed easier and walked silently away. When he reached his house, he went to a chair on the porch. Slowly, taking as much time as he could, ordering his trembling hands to obey him, Reid took out his smokes and lit one, drawing in the first mouthful with a deep hissing inhalation. His only thought was of how beautiful and desirable Heather Strand was.

Chapter Nine

$\mathcal{F}$riday came and brought with it a whirlwind of activity. Because of Emma's absence, Heather worked in the office, taking calls and doing whatever she could. At two o'clock Reid came in from the range and took over. There was ordering and the many other things only he or Emma could handle. With a grateful smile, Heather left the confinement of the office and went to the studio.

Ever since she had awakened this morning she had been anxious to get back to work on Reid's bust. It was like an obsession to finish it as quickly as possible. *Perhaps,* she thought, *when it is finished and fired, some of my feelings will go away.* She wanted to believe that, but the way her heart raced when she thought of him told her the falseness of her thoughts.

Closing the door to the studio, Heather eagerly breathed in the mixed scents of earth and clay that permeated the air. She began to feel even more excitement as she neared her workbench.

First she uncovered the bust. Next she checked the moisture. She had barely been in time. The first edges of dryness were setting in. Heather remonstrated herself for not getting up fifteen minutes earlier to come out and dampen down the clay before starting work in the office. But she had been in time, and that's what counted.

Quickly, Heather filled the porcelain basin with warm water and then used her wet fingers to moisten the clay. Before she started the actual work, she let her fingers "see" Reid's face. She traced his features slowly and almost felt the clay come to life. His full lips, cold in clay, still had the power to burn her fingers. The slight ridge on his nose caused a flicker of a smile on the corner of her lips. His cheekbones, broad and high, matched the arrogance and power that was in his voice. And his eyes, Heather thought as her fingers moved gently over the clay duplicates, were large, well formed, and she knew they would possess both the soft gentleness and the fierce depth she sensed belonged to Reid.

Heather shook her head to clear away her thoughts of the man who had edged so deeply into her mind and heart and began to work with the clay. She smoothed certain areas, refining the angle of his broad jaw before blending in the earlobes until they formed the funny little half-bend that would match Reid's. The mustache had presented her most difficult obstacle, but with patience and a dentist's probe Heather achieved the effect she wanted.

When the mustache was completed, her hands moved to the neck of the bust. Suddenly Heather stopped. Her left hand held the back of the neck. Again the memory of that explosive kiss, when her hand had seemed to move by itself to the back of his neck, flooded her mind. Her fingers began to move in slow circles on the clay, until she stopped at the exact spot where she had touched, that night, a small scar. Until just now, she hadn't remembered it. Using the tips of her first two fingers, Heather pinched a half inch of clay up and, using her fingernail, made the slightest of indentations across the ridge. When she was done, and her fingers told her the scar was right, she nodded in satisfaction.

Once again, Heather explored the clay duplicate of Reid Hunter's face, hair, and neck, even rechecking the small cleft in his chin. When she was finished, she felt a constriction in her throat. She was done. The only thing that remained was the air drying, before putting the sculpture into the kiln.

A sudden wave of fatigue descended on her. Heather's hand automatically went to her watch. She was not surprised to find seven hours had passed since she'd entered the studio. Seven hours of total absorption in what she loved doing the most.

Within ten minutes Heather had straightened up her work area, cleaned the tools she had been using, and checked her specially designed kiln to make sure it was operating properly. With hunger pangs urging her on, she left the studio and went to the house to prepare some supper for herself and to wait out the time until she could put the clay in its oven.

Reid was sitting on the large chair behind the desk, holding the black plastic telephone receiver against his ear and looking out the window. The view from the office was directed at the sculpture-lined walk that led to Heather's studio. Darkness had descended, but the light that was cast from the window illuminated the first three sculptures. As his eyes studied them again, he heard the phone being lifted at the other end.

"Hunter Gallery, good evening," came the familiar sweet voice.

"I tried your apartment, but I won't complain about getting you on the second try."

"Reid," she screamed, and Reid grimaced with the semipain that echoed in his ear. "Where are you?"

"Nevada. The Strand Ranch," he told her.

"It's about time. Don't you think five months is a bit long?" she admonished. Reid felt the old, familiar stirrings of guilt begin.

"There've been longer times," he replied.

"Let's not fight. I miss you. How are you? What are you doing?"

"Slow down," he said, grinning at her staccato questions. "I miss you too. I'm fine, and I'm the foreman here."

"What happened at the Triple-K? I thought you liked it there?"

"Kelly Kingston happened there. She wouldn't take no for an answer," Reid told her, his voice turning serious again.

"The spunky little redhead? I told you so," Gwen said.

"You were right. But that wasn't all of it. I guess I just had to move on," Reid admitted. "It was time."

"Reid, you've been moving on for almost ten years. Don't you think it's time to stop?"

"I made my decision, and I have no plans to change it," he said. But no matter what he told her, nothing he could do stopped the tendrils of sadness from infiltrating his thoughts. "Don't you want to know why I called?" he asked, changing the subject and blocking the old memories before they overtook him.

"I would hope it's because you wanted to hear your little sister's voice," Gwen replied. Reid heard both humor and longing in her tone.

"No one has called you little since you turned fourteen," he joked as the picture of a gangly, freckle-faced tomboy rose in his mind. At fourteen Gwen Hunter had reached the height of five-eight. By seventeen she stood a barefoot five-ten.

"And no one has ever called me stringbean since I was fifteen and you beat the hell out of Richie Compton for saying it."

"I never liked him anyway," Reid said, savoring the memory of the boy's bloody nose.

"Why did you call?" Gwen asked again.

"Partly because I wanted to speak to you, to give you my address, and to find out how you are."

"I'm fine, what's the address, and I'm glad to hear your voice again. When will I see you?"

"I'll probably be able to take a few days at the end of the summer. I'll try to get to Santa Fe," he said.

"You'd better, please."

"Gwen, anything new with the Foundation?"

"Everything's going nicely. We're getting good donations and Mike has set up a camp in the Catskills." Reid nodded as he listened. Mike Bloom was the director of the New Life Foundation and was one of its prime forces.

"That's great. I have news Mike will appreciate. I've set up the groundwork for another camp. I need the paperwork for leasing three hundred acres and a residence. The terms are one dollar annual rental. The

Foundation is responsible for all setup costs. We can use fifteen veterans for the four-month season and a married couple for the year-round custodial work. The camp should accommodate at least forty children. It's what we discussed two years ago." Reid paused. He took a deep breath and then continued. "I also want the lawyer to prepare a loan agreement for The Strand Ranch, Inc., as borrower and the Foundation as lender. The amount is fifty thousand dollars and the interest is six percent."

"Reid! The Foundation doesn't have that much liquid capital for a loan."

"Yes it does. Tell Mike to authorize the loan from the reserve fund that was set up in the beginning."

"Reserve fund? Reid, when did the Foundation get enough money for a reserve fund?" Gwen asked, unable to keep the surprise from her voice.

"I gave it to them."

"Your inheritance?"

"Let it be," he said in a voice filled with warning. He had never told Gwen that when he'd left the ranch he'd given up the trust fund his father had left him as part of his inheritance. Ten years ago, Reid had wanted no part of anything that would remind him of his past life.

"All right," Gwen replied, but Reid heard the reprimand in her voice.

"Gwen, how's . . ." Although he tried, he could not get the name out.

"Patrick's the same as ever," she responded quickly, knowing exactly what Reid was asking.

"The ranch?"

"It's . . . just fine." But Reid heard something in her voice, the hesitation before she finished speaking and something in her tone.

"What's wrong?"

"Nothing," Gwen responded.

"What is wrong?" Reid repeated, clipping each word separately, demanding the truth by his tone.

"I didn't want to say. I'm not sure, but there're problems. I don't know exactly what, but I've heard rumors that Pat's in trouble," Gwen admitted.

"Tell me what you do know," he ordered. Reid's mind was racing, wondering what his brother had done to get one of the most profitable ranches in the Southwest into trouble.

"Chet Downing came to see me. Pat fired him the other day."

"He can't fire Chet," Reid reminded her. In his father's will Chet Downing, the ranch foreman, had been guaranteed a job until he retired, and then would be given an advisory position afterward along with a minor amount of stock.

"Patrick did. Chet told me it was because he argued with Pat about a deal he made. Pat fired him and told him if he didn't like the way he ran the ranch to go someplace else."

"No matter what we think of Pat, he wouldn't intentionally do anything to ruin Broadlands. He couldn't," Reid reminded her.

"Come back and see what's happening," Gwen asked. Her words were almost whispered, but Reid heard them loudly as a cold shock flowed through him.

"No, Gwen. I won't go back."

"Reid, it's been ten years. It's time we were a family again," she said, and Reid heard the tears that were in her voice.

"You and I are our family," he said quietly, then, as he turned the chair and looked out the office window, he saw Heather, accompanied by Polaris, walk into the light cast through the office window.

"Gwen, get the paperwork to me as soon as possible," he said, giving her the address and the telephone number.

"Good-bye, Reid—take care of yourself."

"I'll call again soon," Reid said, ending the call swiftly.

"Don't wait so long next time. I love you," Gwen said softly.

"And I love you too, kid—take care. Say hello to Mike for me." Reid hung up the phone just as the house door closed.

Heather entered through the kitchen door and went directly to the refrigerator. She removed three eggs and took down a stainless steel bowl and a frying pan from the cabinet over the stove. Quickly and efficiently, Heather went about the business of preparing a light supper.

As she filled the coffeepot and put it on the stove, the tangy scent of Reid's tobacco reached her sensitive nostrils. She turned slightly and spoke.

"Hasn't anyone told you it's not polite to stare?" she asked.

"Uh-huh," came his cryptic reply as he stood in the doorway.

"Did you eat yet?"

"Uh-uh."

"Have a seat," she told him as she went to the refrigerator and withdrew more eggs. For some reason his presence had not surprised her. Perhaps, Heather thought abstractly, because of all the time she'd spent working on the sculpture, hearing his voice was like her art coming to life.

"We should have the paperwork for the loan by the end of next week," Reid said. Heather nodded her head in reply, but kept silent. She was enjoying his unexpected company after the long hours of solitude. "I think the . . ."

"Damn! I hear it," she said, moving quickly to the stove and pulling the boiling coffee from the flame. She was upset that she had forgotten to turn down the heat. After a moment, she replaced the pot on the fire and lowered the flame.

"How can you tell how much to reduce the flame?" Reid asked, genuine puzzlement in his voice.

"Close your eyes and listen," Heather told him. Then she lit another burner and listened to the intensity of the high gas flame. "Can you hear that?"

"Uh-huh."

"Now listen," she said as she lowered the flame by two-thirds. "Hear the difference?"

"No," Reid admitted truthfully.

"It takes time," Heather informed him as she turned to smile at him. "Do you want cheese in your eggs?" The question took Reid off guard for a moment.

"However you're having yours will be fine with me."

"Plain," she informed him.

It only took a few minutes for Heather to make the eggs and slip the bread in the toaster. Reid set the table over her protests and poured the coffee as she prepared the rest. They ate silently, enjoying each other's company.

"You make good eggs," Reid said.

"Thank you."

"How's your work coming?"

"I'm almost finished. I'm going to fire it tonight and

by early tomorrow afternoon it will be done," she told him.

"Good," he declared. "Tom tells me you ride," Reid said suddenly.

"Not by myself," Heather told him as a tingle of anticipation began to weave through her mind.

"I'd hoped not."

"I'm a rancher. I have my problems, but I'm still a rancher," she told him smugly.

"I know. Quitting time is around three tomorrow. After I've paid the boys, would you like to take a ride with me?"

"I'd like that very much," Heather said, conscious of the effort it took to keep her voice steady.

"So would I," Reid added. "And Heather, thanks again for supper." Before Heather could reply she heard Reid stand and begin to leave.

"Have a pleasant night," she called to him.

"You too," he said as he closed the screen door behind him.

After several minutes, Heather stood and cleared the table. Then she washed and dried the dishes. Before returning to the studio to fire the clay, Heather called Polaris. She bent slightly and patted her chest. "Give a hug," she said. The dog stood on his hind legs, placing his front paws on her shoulders, and nuzzled her cheek and neck. "Good boy," she cooed as she patted his back. "Okay, run!" she commanded.

Polaris dropped to all fours and gave his single deep bark. Then she heard him turn and walk softly to his door. A moment later she heard the sound of his body as it scraped through the rubber exit. After he was gone, Heather filled a large mug with coffee to bring with her to the studio.

She was tired, yet excited—tired from the long, but

satisfying day, and excited about tomorrow. First would come the clay, then a bath, and then sleep.

And what about you, Reid Hunter? What is it about you that tears me apart and makes me want to reach out and break down those walls that surround you? With a low sigh, Heather left the kitchen and stepped into the pleasant Nevada night.

Chapter Ten

*W*ithin the confines of her bedroom, Heather listened to the coarse jokes the men tossed at each other as they were paid. The Saturday ritual was in full swing, but even the noise and excitement of the men paled in comparison to what Heather was feeling.

Trying to ignore the tension sweeping through her body, Heather concentrated on the men who would very shortly be gone from the ranch. First, they would clean up, dress in their finest clothes, and, no later than four o'clock, be on their way to town. The men who had steady girls would pick them up and take them out to dinner. The other men, who either did not have a girl friend or did not want a steady woman, would eat in twos or threes at a fancy restaurant and afterward hit the honky-tonks, to drink, dance, and hopefully find a willing lady to spend the rest of their time off with.

Heather smiled as she dressed for her ride with Reid. She tucked the blue and yellow plaid Western shirt into the waist of her riding jeans and buckled the wide leather belt. Her finger lingered on the buckle for a moment. It had been her father's. He had given it to her when she had turned fifteen and she always wore it when she rode. Shaking away the memory, Heather picked up one of her riding boots. She ran her fingers across the leather of the Justin boot, feeling the familiar intricacy of the hand-stitched pattern. The leather itself was soft and pliable and felt like the old friend it was.

Heather slipped on the boots and then rolled up the cuffs of her jeans twice. Her anticipation of the ride increased as she heard the first of the cars drive from the ranch's parking lot.

Going to her dresser, Heather picked up the hairbrush and deftly swept her abundant hair back, slipping it into the covered band she held between three opened fingers so her hair would stay behind her shoulders on the ride. Then she felt she was ready. She left the bedroom and walked to the front door.

"Polaris," she called. The dog's answering bark arrived a second before he did. "You're off duty today," she said as she patted his head. "Run!" she commanded. Polaris barked again as he squeezed through the front door ahead of his mistress.

The walk to the stable was short, and Heather answered the cheerful greetings called to her by the departing men. She paused when she reached the stable. The smell of horse and grain was strong, almost, but not quite, covering the fresh scent of *his* aftershave.

"Reid?" she called.

"Over here," came his voice from her left. She turned toward the sound and walked to him. "Tom said you usually ride Savage. Shall I saddle him?" he asked.

"Has he been ridden lately?" Heather asked.

"One of the boys rode fence with him Tuesday. That was the last time."

"Then he should have some exercise, but I'll saddle him if you don't mind."

"It's no trouble," Reid protested, watching Heather walk toward him.

"I like to do for myself," she told him as she stopped in front of the roan gelding's stall and reached out her hand. The horse whinnied as he picked up Heather's scent and brushed against her hand. "Hello, boy," she murmured.

"Your saddle, boss lady," said Reid. Heather wasn't sure of exactly what Reid's tone held besides a slight tinge of resignation. But the electric shock that went through her fingers as their hands met on the saddle wiped the question from her mind.

Five minutes later she led Savage from the stable, holding the reins lightly in her left hand. He had been named by her father, because of the fierce way the gelding stamped his front legs. But it had been a misnomer; Savage was one of the gentlest range horses Heather had ever ridden. He was surefooted and had a light mouth. Just the barest of pressure with the reins was more than enough signal for the horse.

"Ready?" Reid asked as his eyes took in her full figure.

"Can I have a hand?" Heather asked, wanting only to feel his touch on her.

"My pleasure," Reid replied. Heather gripped the pommel as Reid stepped next to her. His hands went to her waist and Heather felt his strength as he lifted her into the saddle. She hadn't needed help to mount since she was ten, but today she wanted some. Then his hands were on her boot, guiding it into the stirrup. She stopped the grin that tried to escape as she quickly slipped her other foot free of the stirrup before he came around the horse.

"Where are we going?" she asked as Reid slipped her other foot into the stirrup and then mounted his horse.

"Anyplace you'd like."

"The old homestead?" she asked.

"Fine," he replied. They started out side by side, Heather listening intently for Reid to set the pace. As they rode—walked, actually—she found herself content to enjoy the late-afternoon sun warming her face.

It was a quarter of an hour later before Heather spoke for the first time. "Let me know when we reach the plateau," she stated. For some reason she knew that Reid was gazing at her intently. "Savage has the smoothest canter of any horse I've ridden," she explained.

"Is there anything you don't do?" Reid asked, keeping his voice as light as possible. He liked the way she sat the horse, her back straight and her seat firm. Her knees were placed lightly against Savage's sides and the reins were held firmly in her right hand. Her left hand rested on her thigh.

"A few things. I don't drive a car."

"Thank the Lord," Reid muttered.

Heather's bubbling laugh flowed from her lips as she reined in the horse. "Thank you, Reid," she said, more seriously, and could not help the emotion that filled her voice.

"For what?"

"For accepting me as I am."

"I haven't had any choice, have I?" he said wryly, without thinking. He knew the words sounded entirely different from what he'd meant.

"You know what I mean."

"I know," he said. "Plateau's over the next rise." Heather felt the anticipation build as they crested the gently sloped hill. She knew the horse felt her excitement by the way his muscles tensed against her thighs.

"We're . . ." she heard Reid begin, but her heels were already against Savage's flanks. The roan whinnied once and began to speed up. Heather sat deeper into the saddle, letting her body sense every movement of the horse, closing off everything around her as she let herself become an extension of the gelding. She moved with Savage, letting her pelvis roll with each stride of the horse. The wind on her face felt as good as the powerful animal beneath her, who cantered smoothly along the grassy plateau.

Heather slowly bent low, never once breaking the rhythm she was in. Pressing her cheek against Savage's neck, she was soon one with the horse. But she did not let her mind lose itself completely, and she heard Reid's horse next to hers. She felt safe, protected, and unafraid.

Reid watched Heather let her horse free. For the first few seconds he held his breath. His breath came back as he watched her, in awe, riding the gelding. There was no doubt in Reid's mind that Heather was a good rider—none at all—as she held the horse in a controlled canter. He used his heels to urge his mount faster, and soon he was next to her. He watched as her body moved expertly with the horse. His eyes roamed along her length and his breath quickened with desire.

Forcefully, Reid brought himself under control. Turning his face forward, he scanned the countryside before them. The edge of the plateau was coming up, and he felt almost saddened that he would have to slow her down.

It might have been five minutes, or five hours, or somewhere in between when she heard Reid's warning call. Regretfully, Heather straightened, gently pulling back on the reins. Savage slowed to a lope, and then to a walk.

Heather sighed. She was aware of the light film of perspiration on her face as she stopped the horse. The barest trickle of salty moisture rolled between her breasts, making her conscious of the work involved in riding a horse. She liked the feeling and the release of tension it always brought with it.

"You ride beautifully," Reid told her. Heather flushed with the compliment.

"I had a good teacher."

"Your father?" he asked.

Heather nodded. "We're almost there, aren't we?" she asked.

"You really know this ranch, don't you." Heather knew it was more a statement than a question.

"I've lived . . ."

". . . here all my life," Reid finished for her.

Heather nodded as another bubbly laugh surfaced. "Besides, the homestead is only a half-mile from the plateau," she explained. Then she paused, a strong desire filling her mind. "Reid, tell me what you see."

Reid looked at the blue-eyed woman who was next to him and at the open, longing expression that filled her face. But, strangely, he was not saddened by her request, only glad she asked.

"I see beauty." Heather heard the depth of emotion that carried in his voice. "Off to our left must be the granddaddy of this part of the Sierra Nevada—it's the tallest mountain in sight. Its face is green, right up to the timberline, and there's still some snow left on its peak. The colors of the trees are deep, but there's a lot of shading. The homestead is off to the right, but we can't see it from here."

Reid paused for a moment, trying to put into words what he was seeing and feeling.

"Right below us is more level ground, sagebrush, Indian rice grass, and plenty of trees there too, but not like on the big mountain—small pines and some magnificent aspens, lots of cedar on the low slopes, kind of a grayish green."

Heather heard Reid take another breath before he continued.

"The trees and the grass are only part of it. It's more than just color—it's space, and freedom, and I guess the biggest part is the peace. I mean, it's open, quiet, and free."

"I think I understand," Heather told him, touched by his expressiveness.

"And it will be appreciated by the kids who will be here next year."

"Tell me about them," she prompted as they began to ride down from the plateau.

"They're beautiful," Reid said, still caught up in the emotions of the countryside. "Most of the children the Foundation helps are the children of Vietnamese refugees who have fled their homes."

"Boat people?" Heather asked softly.

"Some. Most are the ones that got away in the last days before Saigon fell. But all the children aren't Asian—they're a mixture of Vietnamese and American veterans' kids. Most people have forgotten about the men who fought in the war."

"It's been a while since it ended," Heather offered.

"Only for those who weren't there. Here we are,"

Reid said suddenly, changing the direction the conversation had taken as he stopped the horses fifty feet from the old homestead house.

"I laid out the boundaries last Sunday. When the Foundation starts work, they'll put up a fence completely around the camp. Work on the homestead will start in the spring, and by June everything will be ready."

"Don't you ever take a day off?" Heather joked.

"Once a year or so," Reid responded.

"I can believe that," Heather said, and for some reason she did.

"Want to walk a bit?"

"Love to," Heather replied. She dropped Savage's reins over his head, the signal the horse had been taught when he was supposed to stand still. Lithely, Heather slipped her right foot from the stirrup and began to dismount. As her leg crossed over the saddle, she felt Reid's hands at her waist, steadying her. Reid lowered her to the ground and her back slid along his chest. Again her body's instant reaction to his took her by surprise. Her breath caught in her throat, and she stood tensely for a moment until she recovered. Only then did she turn.

Heather felt Reid take her elbow and begin to guide her. It took a few moments to adjust to the ground— her legs still felt the breadth of the horse.

"The training corral will be here," Reid began as he explained the layout of the camp. Although she listened to his words and understood everything he was saying, something else held her attention. The something else was his hand on her arm and the melodious sound of his voice. For the first time since she'd met Reid Hunter, Heather quieted her internal war and began to simply enjoy his presence. She had no idea how long a time they walked for, nor did she care. Every concern and every worry she'd had seemed to have been soothed away by his voice.

Then, suddenly, his next words shattered her mood. "We should be heading back now. Tom wants to leave by six and I don't want to leave the ranch shorthanded."

Heather's fingers automatically went to the watch face and she realized that they had been out for over two hours. It was five thirty. "I almost forgot," she said, recalling that Tom and Gregg were driving to Carson City tonight so that Gregg could go to the rodeo on Sunday. Turning quickly, she bumped into Reid. "Sorry," she mumbled, his heady male scent making her heart pound loudly. She was very aware of his hands on her shoulders and of her legs threatening to turn into rubber.

Reid was unable to move out of the way of her sudden turn and his hands instinctively went to her shoulders to steady her. He looked down into her face and froze. He was aware of the heat of her skin on his hands rising through the fabric of her shirt. He was conscious of her breasts pressed against his chest and of the way the sun brought out fiery highlights as it played on her hair. His mouth turned suddenly dry, and he was having trouble breathing. "Heather," he whispered.

She heard him call her name, but it was a sound made distant by the racing of her blood and the spinning of her head. She felt her arms go around his back and she lifted up on her toes. Her lips met his and a flaming, lancing fire raced through her body. She felt his hands dig into her shoulders as his mouth pressed forcefully against hers. Her lips opened and she tasted his tongue as it searched for hers. Everything in her world of sound and touch receded except for the feel of Reid against her.

For Reid, time stood still as he pressed Heather to him. His need burned deeply, and for the first time in ten years he knew he wanted someone with his heart and his mind, not just with his body. Yes, he felt the desire for Heather flooding him, but the desire was encased by something different, something that gave him the ability to understand what was happening, and to regret it. This was the first time he realized what he had given up ten years ago.

"Heather . . ." he said again, hearing the harshness of his own voice sound unbearably loud in his ears.

"No!" Heather said as his mouth left hers and she heard him speak her name. She did not realize she'd spoken aloud as her hands pulled away from his back. One hand went to his face, to trace along his cheek. She felt sadness in her fingertips and understood how much the single word had cost Reid.

She took a deep, shuddering breath as she slowly withdrew her hand. She turned from him and walked several steps away. "You must think I'm terrible," she whispered, images of wanton women from the stories she'd heard parading through her thoughts.

"You're anything but terrible," Reid said as he walked up behind her. He put a hand on her shoulder and watched as one of hers covered it. The softness of her skin and its gentle heat made him swallow several times before he could continue. "I only wish . . ." he began, again searching for the right words.

"That you didn't believe in what you believe in? I don't think you'd be half the man you are if that were the case," Heather told him in a low voice, pressing his hand with hers. Stepping back, she forced a smile to her lips as she faced him.

"Wanna race back?" she asked in mock challenge, fighting away the helplessness of her feelings and at the same time trying to make up for again placing Reid at the disadvantage.

"No, thanks—I don't like to lose."

"Chicken!"

"Yes, ma'am," Reid agreed. He gazed at her, watching her face, but was unable to read the expression that was there. He took her arm again and led her back to the horses. As he was about to help her up, he saw Heather grasp the pommel and pull herself neatly into the saddle. Then he smiled, thinking about when he had helped her mount at the stable.

"And don't 'Yes, ma'am' me!" she ordered as she sat proudly on the horse's back.

"Yes, ma'am," Reid replied.

The ride back was as pleasant as the ride out. Neither mentioned the incident at the old homestead, and to Heather it seemed as if it had only been a figment of her imagination. Her regret was that it seemed to take almost no time at all to return to the stable.

When they reached the ranch, Tom and Gregg had already left. There were two men on duty tonight and Sunday besides Reid, and after she and Reid unsaddled and brushed and watered their horses, Reid joined the other men for dinner and Heather went to her own house alone.

The first thing she did was to take a frozen pot pie and put it in the oven. Then, feeling the muscles of her thighs begin to tighten from the unaccustomed length of the ride, she ran hot water into the tub and, while it was filling, undressed.

Emitting a deep, heartfelt sigh of gratitude, Heather slipped into the bath. It had been a long day, but vastly different from the day before. From early this morning until she turned on the water for her bath, Heather had not stopped for more than five minutes at a time.

She could feel the hot water working its magic beneath the layers of her skin. The soothing and gentle heat drew the fatigue from her muscles and Heather felt her mind and body become separate entities. The scented bath oil she had liberally used coated her skin with a delicious silkiness that further added to her comfort.

Slowly Heather began to knead her thigh in an effort to force her protesting muscles to loosen. A smile played on her lips as she thought about the day.

The morning had been perfect, filled with activity and satisfaction. By noon Reid's clay bust had cooled, and she had examined it minutely to make sure the firing process had been perfect. It had, and she had been relieved. Heather's biggest worry when working with firing clay had been the final process. Because she was blind, she could not check on the work as it was being heated and then cooled. Even with the special computer modifications that automatically set the temperatures and checked on the clay's progress, the procedure had always been a slow torture until Heather could actually "see" the finished piece.

Heather sighed as she moved her hands to her other thigh and began to manipulate the muscles. She remembered again, vividly, her sensation of pleasure with the finished bust. It had been a very different feeling than she had had when she'd completed one of her other pieces. Usually some depression came with the completion of a work, but today another reaction had overtaken her. It had been a feeling that was a combination of the satisfaction of a job well done and the excitement of the knowledge that she would be spending the afternoon with the living, talking, and animated version of what her hands had been holding.

As Heather's thigh muscles relaxed, she sank lower in the tub. Only then did she allow herself to think about what had happened at the homestead. The kiss they had shared. Heather realized it had not been like the first one, so many weeks ago. The suddenness of its intensity had robbed her of her will. Her entire body had surrendered to his, and she had been unable to prevent it. She also realized, belatedly, that she had sensed a similar response in Reid. Only he had been strong and had stopped himself.

She also learned something else today about Reid. Emma Kline was right. Reid was not your average cowboy, not even your above-average foreman. He spoke too well, too eloquently. He bared feelings that she would never have expected when he spoke about the land and, even more so, when he spoke of the camp and the children.

I've learned something about myself, too, Heather admitted. *I've learned that I'm capable of making a fool of myself.* For the first time since she'd met Reid, Heather understood what was happening to her. She had never in her life, ever, just bumped into someone. She had an unexplained form of radar that always let her know where the people around her were. It was a sense she had developed and one that had never failed her. It hadn't today; she had just ignored it and ended up in Reid's arms. *He must think me a perfect fool,* she thought, and felt embarrassed at her earlier, seemingly wanton actions. *Why am I acting like this? Why does Reid affect me this way?* she wondered again, as she had almost every day recently.

Shaking her head, Heather bent forward and opened the tub's drain. She stood and reached for the large terry bath sheet, and as she stepped from the tub she wrapped herself in its softness.

After she dried herself, Heather applied powder and put on a bathrobe. She slid her feet along the carpet, searching for her slippers until she remembered she hadn't brought them in.

"Polaris," she called. A moment later she heard the dog come into the bathroom. "Slippers," she told him. Less than a minute later, Polaris dropped the slippers at her feet. "Good boy," she said as she put them on.

Heather felt hungry then and went to the kitchen to check the oven timer. Barely an hour had passed since she'd put the frozen chicken pie in the oven. She had another few minutes before it would be ready. It was enough time to dress, she decided as she walked to her bedroom. She chose a soft white cotton dress that covered her and flowed smoothly from her neck to her ankles. Discarding her slippers, Heather put on a pair of leather-tong sandals. Then she deemed herself ready for dinner.

Dinner had been good, but lonely, Heather thought as she placed a cassette in the tape deck and sat back comfortably on the couch. A few seconds later, John Denver's voice floated in the air.

I'm lonely, Heather thought, *because of the time this afternoon I spent with Reid.* Now it seemed like the ride had been months ago, instead of hours. She had enjoyed being with him. She had more than just enjoyed it, Heather admitted to herself. Much more.

Listening to the refrains of "Rocky Mountain High," she thought of the talk she and Emma had had the other night. Emma's story had affected her deeply, and she knew that it had not been easy for Emma to speak of her past. Heather had always suspected something, but until the older woman actually told her she had not been sure.

Suddenly Heather stood. Without understanding how, she reached a decision about her life. Striding purposefully to the stereo, she turned it off. Then she walked to the front door, opened it, and stepped outside.

Heather sniffed the air and scented moisture. Maybe a rain shower, she thought as she descended the front steps. On the ground, she paused as a chill rushed across her skin, a chill the coolness of the late-night mountain air had not caused. Then, with a deeply drawn breath, she began to walk toward the small house Reid Hunter occupied.

A tremor passed through her hands and she knew how nervous she was. She'd never done anything like this before, but she knew if she was not the one to act, if it was not she who took her destiny into her own hands, she might lose something that was very, very important to her. She might lose the love she now knew had been growing steadily within her heart.

She was going to do what she had to. She was going to confront the man responsible, and one way or another, something would be settled tonight.

Chapter Eleven

*R*eid paced the confines of his small living room. The energy that possessed him made him feel like a caged animal. His reflection in the window made him pause and grin. He looked like one, too. He wore only his jeans. His bare chest, with its mat of curly hair, looked as menacing in the glass as did the scowl that had been on his face.

After the ride this afternoon, he had eaten dinner with the two men who were on weekend duty and afterward had driven to the north range to check on the foals that had been let loose there yesterday. Everything had been all right and he had returned by ten. It was now almost midnight, but Reid did not want to go to bed. After what had happened today with Heather, he knew he would not be able to sleep very well.

Reid paused in his pacing and thought again about Heather Strand. He knew she was a strong woman, but at the same time he realized her vulnerability and her inexperience. What was obvious to him was the fact that her emotions were telling him a story that he was afraid to listen to. He was afraid, he admitted, because if he let his guard down for even an instant, his own repressed emotions would burst forth, a mirror image of Heather's, and he knew that that could not be allowed to happen.

It couldn't happen because ten years ago he'd given up the ability to be on equal terms with Heather Strand, when he'd given up his rights, and money, in order to change what his life had become. Reid also knew there could be no future for Heather and himself on that unequal basis—his pride would not allow it.

"Damn!" he muttered as he sank into a chair. No good. Reid stood and walked to the window. He froze as he saw a billowy form change from a shadow into a walking ghost. No, it was Heather Strand in a white dress, walking in his direction.

Reid watched, fascinated, as she approached. She was like a softly moving vision, her footsteps secure as she moved inexorably, he realized suddenly, toward this very house. She came nearer and, as the light from his porch reached her face, Reid saw the determination that filled her. A moment later she disappeared from sight. Then he heard the low knock on his door.

"Reid?" her voice called softly. Five steps were all that was necessary for him to reach the door and open it.

"Is something wrong?" he asked.

"Yes. Invite me in."

"You're invited," he told her as he stepped back.

Heather felt her pulse race as she stepped inside his house. Her senses reeled under the assault of Reid's living quarters: the smell of tobacco, of the old furniture, and, above all, of Reid himself attacked her every step.

"What's wrong?" he asked, concerned that something bad had brought her here at this late hour.

"Us," she said.

"Us?" he echoed, stunned by her words. "Heather, there is no us."

"There is. Reid, please don't make this hard, but I've got to say what's on my mind." Heather paused, her heart beating wildly as she waited for Reid to say something, anything. But, of course, he didn't—just as she had known he wouldn't. "You're making this difficult."

"It's not difficult, it's impossible," Reid said, knowing he had no choice, hurting inside as he watched her. Then he saw her face change. The uncertainty that had been in it a bare second before was gone. In its place was determination.

"Will you be honest with me?" Heather asked. Concentrating on his reply, Heather willed her mind to see his words.

"I don't want to hurt you," he said in a low voice.

"Will you be honest?" she repeated.

"Yes."

Heather heard the truth as he spoke the single word. "You're a difficult man, Reid Hunter—difficult, honest, and troubled." Heather paused to take a deep preparatory breath, filling her lungs with the scent of him. "But you're still a man, and one with feelings." Heather waited knowing there could be no turning back now.

Reid, too, knew he must reply this time. He looked at her and felt the longing and desire try to break free. He forced the emotions down and found it was the hardest task he'd undertaken in the last ten years. "I'm your foreman, Heather. I work for you and you need me here. You need me to keep this ranch alive, to bring it back up to the level your father had reached. You can't sacrifice that—you can't!" Even as he spoke, Reid was aware of the desperation in his voice.

"Must we sacrifice something more important?" she asked.

"This ranch is what's important," Reid told her bluntly.

"Do you believe that?" Heather asked in a whisper.

To Reid's ears the whisper was a roar. "I have to, for both of us."

"Reid, I found out something today—something very important. The ranch is only land—you and I are people. I don't care what anyone else has to say."

"You don't have any choice! We don't have any choice," Reid said, realizing he'd admitted what she had said was true.

"The rules of the cowboy?" she said bitterly. This was going wrong, Heather thought. He was avoiding the issue and making her feel like a fool.

"It's more than just that."

"Is it what happened to you in the war?" Heather asked suddenly. Some deep-down intuitive process told her to probe, and she did not question why.

"That has nothing to do with this ranch," Reid replied, but even he heard the lie in his voice.

"You're here, and it's because of certain things that have happened to you. Reid, I know you have feelings for me. I can sense them and you can't deny them. But instead of doing something about those feelings, you hide behind some antiquated creed and say that you're protecting me. I came here because of the way I feel about you—don't make me any more ashamed of what I'm doing than I already am."

Reid felt his throat tighten as he looked at her. He

knew then how brave she was, how much this talk and her admission had cost her. And he, too, accepted some of the shame for what was happening, the shame of watching a person he cared for humble herself. He stepped up to her and took her hand in his. He noticed the way it trembled and pressed it tightly as he spoke.

"A lot happened to me in the war and I can't talk about it to anyone—I haven't been able to. But I've learned to live with it. I've made my own sort of peace. But you have to remember that I am your foreman, and in order to make this ranch function the way it should, I have to stick to the rules," Reid said, speaking honestly, believing fully in what he said. "You live in the middle of ranching territory and you must deal with the other ranch owners around you. You need them also, and having an . . . an affair with your foreman will affect your relationship with them."

"You're wrong," she stated.

"Heather, the first time I saw you, when you were in the studio with Gregg, something happened to me. I've been fighting it ever since. I know what the results will be, and it can't be allowed. If something were to happen between us, I know I'd end up hurting you and the ranch. I don't want that to happen," Reid admitted.

"I'm a big girl, and I can play by the rules. I'll live two lives if that's what it takes for us to have a little happiness. Reid, I've never felt anything like what I have since I met you. I've tried to avoid it, to stop it from happening, but I can't. And today I found out I don't want to. Reid, I learned something important today at the homestead."

Reid watched her face, holding her still trembling hand within his. He knew what her next words would be and closed his eyes as she spoke.

"I learned that what I've been fighting cannot be

fought. To fight is to lose. I learned that I love you. No!" Heather said quickly, cutting off the reply that she knew was coming. "Don't say anything. Please, Reid, just hold me."

Reid released her hand and drew her into his arms. He pressed her to his bare chest and felt the dampness on her cheek mingle with the hair of his chest. He held her tightly against him for an eternity, until at last he bent down and lifted her face to his.

Heather's tears flowed as she buried her face against his warmth. She had said it. She had told him. Now there was nothing else to say or do. But against him, now, she was safe. The heat of his body and the security of his arms held her dark world at bay. She had been completely honest, and in doing so she had unleashed a raw depth of emotions she had not known she possessed.

Slowly, Reid's hand moved up her back and cupped her head. She felt him draw her head back and then felt his lips on hers. There were no lancing fires, no explosions of desire, only the gentle soft warmth of his mouth on hers. She returned the kiss, aware of the teary saltiness in her mouth but uncaring at the same time. There were no words, only feelings, only the sounds of their breathing and their hearts as they began to beat together.

Heather felt herself being lifted. The sensation of floating securely within Reid's arms was dizzying as she again buried her face in his chest. She was aware of his movement and of the power and strength of the arms that held her. She could hear the heavy beating of his heart in her ear as he walked from the living room. Soon she felt herself placed on the down quilt of Reid's bed.

Again she was almost overwhelmed by the scent of

the man. It permeated the linens and the room itself. She felt Reid sit next to her on the bed. She reached out her arms and Reid entered her embrace. Her hands were on his back and she pulled him against her. Their mouths met again and she tasted him. Their tongues danced as their breathing grew strained. His hands explored her body as hers continued to play along his back. Every muscle, every hair became a part of her odyssey, and she reveled in the feel of him. Suddenly his fingers were at the zipper of her dress. She felt and heard, simultaneously, the dress being opened. Reid drew the dress down to her waist, exposing her to his eyes. After a moment's anguished wait, Heather felt the burning brand of his lips on her shoulder. Then she was floating again as Reid's hands began to explore her body. When his fingers reached her breasts, she felt herself shudder. When his lips replaced his hands, she cried out. Her fingers went to his hair, weaving through it, feeling the thick waves as if it were a part of herself.

"Love me, Reid, please love me," she whispered in the deafening silence of the bedroom. She felt Reid leave the bed. In the quiet of the room she heard him undressing. A moment later he returned and his hands went to the dress that was at her waist. With her help he slid it completely free.

His sharply indrawn breath shattered the night and she too held her breath.

"You're beautiful, Heather, so beautiful," Reid said in a voice filled with desire as he gazed at Heather. His blood raced madly through him as his eyes hungrily devoured her. From her face to her feet, Heather was a picture of perfection to him. Her skin shined in the low light cast through the bedroom doorframe. The rise and fall of her breasts was an invitation that could not be ignored. The subtle curves of her body called to him, and no longer did any thought of the consequences of the night enter his mind. His thoughts were so filled with the wonder and the vision of the woman he wanted that nothing else could intrude.

Slowly, almost reverently, Reid joined Heather on the bed. He kissed her forehead, trailing his lips across the tanned skin until they found her closed eyelids. His mouth caressed the lids and then wandered along her cheek until he reached her lips. His hands caressed her shoulders, dropping slowly to cover the soft mounds of her breasts. He felt the heat and warmth and let his eyes feast on her beauty.

Heather felt him join her again, felt his lips on her skin, skipping along her forehead, across her eyes, and finally his lips meeting hers. Every sense was alive. She could feel herself vibrate at his every touch and could feel the outpouring of heat from his body as it grazed along hers.

His hands caressed her shoulders, sending shivers of anticipation through her body. Heather almost cried out when his gentle hands reached her breasts. Then she knew she was crying again, silently, because of the love she felt for this big, gentle man, who caressed her so lovingly.

His lips were on her neck, and the desire she had been holding back suddenly exploded within her. She pressed her body to his and heard a low moan float in the air above her. Hazily, she realized it was her own. Then she felt his lips burn a path from her shoulder to the valley between her breasts. She bit her lip at the instant his mouth surrounded the awaiting tip of her breast. All the while her hands wove patterns in his hair until she could no longer restrain the needs that cried out within her.

"Reid," she whispered as she drew his head from her

breast and brought his lips to hers. They kissed. Heather's fingers explored his face, touching his eyes softly, tracing the outline of his ears, stroking his cheeks, until she felt him pull away slightly.

He returned quickly, covering her body with his, fitting his larger, wider frame perfectly on hers. She felt small, dwarfed by his size above her but safe. Her hands were again on his back, kneeding the finely etched muscles, exploring as much of him as she could reach. Slowly she felt Reid move, and she moved also, fitting herself around him.

Heather felt Reid's hands move under her and lift her slightly. She felt him come to her, felt him enter her with love and gentleness. And they were making love.

Heather was carried aloft, feeling sensations she had never known before. She was aware, totally, of everything that was happening. Every movement he made seemed to radiate throughout her entire being. Every breath he took she heard and felt. He was everywhere within her body and within her mind. The desire she had thought so strong before multiplied, driving away all rational thought, leaving only the sensation that the two of them were alone in the universe.

Heather was sure of only one thing—that she loved Reid Hunter fully. There were no doubts now as he carried her to a place she had never known before. Her senses were magnified as she floated higher and higher, until she reached unimaginable peaks.

And then, after a lifetime, she was back.

Her head was cradled between Reid's neck and shoulder, her breath harsh but beginning to slow. She felt Reid's hands running along her back, soothing her, comforting her, helping her. She moved her mouth from the skin on his shoulder to his lips and kissed him slowly.

"I never knew . . ." she began. Reid stopped her with another gentle kiss. Reluctantly, she felt Reid turn onto his side and pull her with him. He kissed her forehead as he wrapped his arms around her. Heather nestled against him, content with the silence, glad for it, and drew on the strength and warmth of her lover.

Reid held her tightly, waiting for his mind to settle and for some semblance of sanity to return. Even as he held Heather close, he could not stop the memory of what had happened only moments ago. He had made love to her and had felt things that he had thought impossible. Just her fingers tracing along his face had sent his desires soaring to heights he'd not been able to contain. The feel of her skin against his, the touch of her hands on his back, and the look of her face as he made love to her had all combined to make him forget everything except the two of them. And it had been wonderful.

Reid smelled her hair, burying his mouth and nose within it. His hands held her close as the heat again began to rise on her skin. Slowly, he turned Heather onto her back and began to caress her. They kissed, and he savored the sweetness of her lips for a long moment.

This time they made love slowly, moving in a perfect rhythm as they learned more about each other. They flew again to infinite heights before returning to earth and the comfort of each other's arms. Content and satisfied, they drifted off to sleep together.

Heather woke slowly and felt the comfort of Reid's arm still around her. She lay still and smiled. They had made love and she had indeed learned she had been right. She was in love with him, as she had told him. And even though he had not said so, every action, every move he had made convinced her he loved her, too. Carefully, so as not to disturb him, Heather lifted Reid's arm and left the bed. When she stood, she waited to make sure he had not awakened.

Slowly, Heather slipped to the floor and searched for her dress. She found it and put it on. She knew that it would be morning soon—she could tell by the air—and she wanted to be gone before Reid awoke. She was now committed to his rules. She had known this before she reached Reid's house and promised herself she would obey. Quietly Heather went to the far side of the bed and bent. She reached out until she felt his hair. Slowly, with the lightest of touches, she traced his lips.

"Good night, my love," she whispered as she straightened and turned. Very carefully, so as not to bump into anything, Heather left the bedroom. Once in the living room, where she had been a frequent visitor when Hank Thompson had been foreman, she moved quickly and left the house. Outside, as she walked toward her house, she felt something furry brush her leg.

"Hi, boy," she said to Polaris. The dog pressed gently against her calf as he led her home.

Chapter Twelve

*H*eather woke with a start. The sound of a car engine echoed loudly in her ears. She listened for a moment as her heart slowed. Each sound held meaning for Heather. This sound was Reid's Land-Rover. She lay still for a moment as she listened to the vehicle's engine fade into the distance.

Slowly, Heather willed her body to move. She had slept late—she knew that without even checking her clock. When she did, she learned it was ten. But rather than rising, Heather stayed within the comfort of her bed and let her mind wander. She could still feel the many sensations that had overwhelmed her last night— the gentle yet firm caresses that Reid had showered her with; the way he held her, and the fires he had ignited.

When she had left Reid last night and walked what seemed the endless distance between his place and hers, she had immediately blocked out her emotions, suddenly afraid of what she had so brazenly started.

But Heather knew she could not deny that this morning her world had been changed irrevocably, and in the new world she had awakened to, Heather Strand had become a different person. Last night she had said what she felt she must and she had meant every word. She had listened to Reid's logical words and then she had acknowledged her love to Reid, knowing she would accept the sacrifices that were part of that growing love. But now, as the memory of his caresses returned with a burning force she had not thought possible, her promises seemed like insignificant shouts in the face of a brewing storm.

Briefly, Heather wondered what had happened to her once firm resolve that she would never again allow a man to enter her heart, to hurt and cause her pain. *But I started it this time,* she told herself firmly, *and I'll see it through.*

Pushing her thoughts aside, Heather rose and went to the bathroom. She stepped into the shower and let the steaming water run over her skin, chasing away the last shadows of sleep. When she was dry and dressed, she made a pot of coffee and went to the studio. She wasn't hungry and skipped breakfast. She had work to do today, and she knew, too, that she needed to keep her mind occupied. Heather refused to allow herself to dwell on last night's events.

Heather worked furiously, making the mold for the first casting of the sculpture of Reid's head. It would take a full twenty-four hours before the plaster dried completely. When it had, she would separate the two halves and begin the process she preferred above all others. After the plaster casts were finished she would use them as a mold to make yet another cast of the sculpture, this time in wax. Once the wax bust was done, she would make her final decision on casting it—whether to cast the metal directly in the plaster, making two halves that would be welded together, or use the lost-wax method. Heather preferred the lost-wax method because it required no welding (she, of course, could not do the welding herself) and to use the plaster-cast method would mean trusting her work to another's hands. When she used the lost-wax method, she had one of the ranch hands help her pour the molten metal into the cast, but her hands were there also.

Heather shook her head. She knew she had already made up her mind. It would be she, with someone's assistance, who would pour molten metal into a frame that encased the wax sculpture. When it cooled, the bronze would replace the wax that had been there. But that, thought Heather, was weeks away.

By two o'clock Heather could no longer ignore the hunger pangs that rippled through her body. With a sigh of acceptance, she finished pouring the last of the plaster and washed her hands. Drying them with the towel, Heather took another deep breath and left the studio.

She made herself lunch and, eating in the living room, listened to the stereo in an effort to avoid thinking about Reid. Finally she gave in and let her mind again replay the events of the previous night. When she was through, she felt a great weight leave her shoulders and realized that she had been fooling herself. She could not fight what her mind told her was right, but neither would she break the promise she had made to Reid. She would play by the rules, no matter what her personal cost might be.

Sighing with resignation, Heather took a sip of lukewarm coffee. She tried to figure out what she could do for the rest of the afternoon. Usually she spent it working in the studio or doing something with Tom and Gregg. Heather smiled as she thought of the young boy. He was so innocent, so filled with fun, that she still found it hard to believe his mother had left him.

Just then the CB base in the office came to life. Hearing Reid's voice fill the air, Heather stood and, with the half cup of coffee still in one hand, moved gracefully through the living room and into the office, where she went to a table against the far wall. On the table was the ranch's CB base station. With a practiced movement, Heather lifted the microphone and pressed the transmitter switch.

"Strand base," she said, and then released the switch.

"Rover One," came Reid's voice again.

"Reid, where are you?" she asked.

"At the homestead. I wanted to check in to make sure everything is all right. Any problems?" he asked.

Heather took a deep breath, forcing the fast beating of her heart to slow. Were there any problems? Is water wet? she wanted to say. "Everything is quiet around here," she said instead.

"How are you?" Reid asked suddenly. Again Heather felt a flutter in her chest.

"F-fine," she replied.

"Good. I'll be in within the hour," he told her as he signed off. Heather cleared the channel, then stood silently in thought.

She wanted very badly to hear his voice in person. She needed to touch him, if just for an instant, to prove to herself that what happened last night was not a cruel dream invading the privacy of her sleep. With that thought Heather crossed the room and went into her office. She wanted to sit in her father's chair and think. Heather knew she still had a lot to think about, a lot to understand.

Sitting in her father's old chair, she tried to draw comfort from its accustomed feel as if it were an old friend. Her fingers would not stay still as they explored the soft leather and suddenly Heather could almost imagine her father here with her. But again she was unsuccessful at avoiding the things she most wanted to escape from—the combination of thoughts that continually ran into each other, careening madly in the intricate maze her mind was fast turning into.

There was the old, always explosive collision of the obligation she was tied to—the Strand Ranch—which fought against her desire to immerse herself totally in her art. But today the old battle of logic against emotion had an added feature. Reid Hunter.

Once again Heather found herself thinking about the ruggedly handsome, mustached man she had shared herself with. Suddenly the quiet of the ranch and the need to try and cleanse herself of the shadowy guilt she felt forced Heather into a deeper contemplation of what had really happened last night.

What had possessed her to be so forward? Reid must think her no more than a common hussy, the way she had acted. She had never done anything like it before and she herself hadn't exactly known what she was going to do when she reached his door last night.

Taking a deep, shuddering breath, Heather willed her mind to become calm. Realistically, she knew there was nothing she could do about what happened last night. She also acknowledged it had been she, not Reid, who had forced the issue. But what would happen now?

The rumble of the Land-Rover's engine pulled

Heather from her thoughts. Again she felt her heart skip a beat. Realizing that nothing within her mind could be resolved at this point, Heather reminded herself of her promise to Reid, forcing away the desire to be held by him from her thoughts as she waited for him.

Moments later, Reid's footsteps resounded in the front office. They stopped, and Heather heard him call her name.

"In here," she replied. Reid's steps picked up again and grew louder in her ears until they stopped across the desk from her.

"'Afternoon," he said. The silence that followed his greeting hung heavily between them until Heather wanted to scream. "Did you sleep at all last night?"

"Do I look that bad?" she asked with a smile. "I slept until I heard you drive away."

"Good. No, you look wonderful," Reid told her as the longing that had been with him all day grew even stronger. He tried to push it aside, to thrust it into that special place he had within him, as he had done successfully with all his emotions since returning from Vietnam. But at this moment he seemed to have lost that hard-earned ability. "About last night . . ." he began.

His words sent a cry of agony through her mind. *Touch me! Hold me! Kiss me!* her heart yelled silently. "The night was ours—the day belongs to the ranch. It's your way. I agreed." Reid studied her carefully and saw the taut set of her mouth and heard the clipped way she spoke. He knew how much those words had cost her, were costing her. He knew all too well.

"You're a magnificent lady, Heather Strand," he told her in a strained voice.

"But dumb!" she replied, forcing a soft lilt into her voice.

"No, blind." Heather laughed at Reid's bantering reply, understanding immediately the joking way he had meant it.

"I meant stupid," she said after another moment of silence. But this time Heather was unable to put the light, lilting tone into her words. The sudden explosion of Reid's hand on the desk top made Heather jump. Polaris, hidden behind the chair, rose quickly to all fours, growling deep in his throat as he moved protectively next to his mistress.

"Don't ever say anything like that again," Reid told her in a hoarse voice. "Not to me. Not to anyone!"

"Reid . . ." She whispered his name. Heather tried to stop the moisture that his deeply felt words brought to her eyes. Her hand went to Polaris's head to calm and reassure the dog.

"I'm sorry, Heather, but I won't listen to you put yourself down. Not you." Reid stopped himself before he had added the word *too*. When Heather had said those last words, a picture of his sister had grown in his mind. She had said the same thing to him six years ago. Gwen had told him she was stupid, stupid to have fallen in love. And Reid knew, even though Heather hadn't said it, that she had meant the same thing.

Reid moved quickly around the desk and pulled Heather to her feet. Her breath left her in a sudden sigh as he crushed her against his chest. He held her there, tightly, without moving. She felt the rise and fall of his chest and the way his heart beat within it. She was afraid to move, yet she knew she could not stay there. Slowly, painfully, she pulled away.

"Tell me about the foals," she said, desperately

trying to ease the charged tension that was between them.

"They're fine," he said to her as he forced himself to think about the seven foals that had been born over the last three weeks. "I think they'll make good dude stock," he said, referring to the type of horses they sold to the resort ranches throughout the Southwest. "But I think we'll do a lot better soon," he finished as he walked back around the desk and sat at the same time as Heather.

"It's still going to take a while, even after we get the new studs."

"I'm working on that also. I've got a few ideas in mind," Reid said as his body unwound. The tension of a few moments ago began to drain away along with the instant desire that had flared so suddenly.

"Such as?" Heather asked, throwing herself fully into the conversation.

"Have you ever considered cattle?" he asked.

"Father had once, but he felt the expenses wouldn't warrant the small profits. We're too far from the major shipping points. We'd have to ship them by truck and the profit would be eaten up," she said as she remembered clearly the discussions she had heard between her father and Hank Thompson.

"He was right, but he was also thinking in much larger terms than I am. I'm thinking of Tahoe, Reno, and northern California. If we can get good beef, undersell the Texas, Dakota, and Kansas markets to the local distributors, we can build a small, but good profit reserve in order to strengthen our main business— horses. Let me play with it a while, boss lady, and I'll see how viable it is," he finished.

But Reid had already been thinking about it. He had

even put out some feelers. If his idea worked out, the money that came from the cattle would support the breeding and raising of a higher grade horse stock. And that was what the Strand Ranch was all about. But even if his plan worked out, he knew, they were still several years away from his goal.

"You're my foreman, the general manager of the Strand Ranch. Do what you think is best," Heather told him flatly, meaning every word she said. It was what she had promised him when he had been hired. Feeling a need for movement, Heather pushed herself from the desk and stood. She walked around the desk to where Reid was seated. She could sense him, a bare inch from her. Her heart was racing again and she knew he could read her desire.

The warmth of his hand as it gripped hers made Heather's breath catch in her throat, but she forced herself to behave normally. Heather realized his hand on hers was as welcome as would be his lips. She smiled at him and spoke again. "But since you've shown just how good a foreman you are, you've shamed me into understanding that I'm going to have to pay more attention to the ranch and less to my hobby," she said, withdrawing her hand.

"Hobby?" Reid repeated, and Heather heard the question in the single word.

"Sculpturing."

"What you do, Heather, is by no means a hobby. Why haven't you had a show yet?" Reid asked the question in a quiet way, but Heather knew he would brook nothing less than the truth.

"I can't yet," she said in a low voice.

Can't, or won't? Reid thought, but this time he held his tongue. "Why?"

"It takes a lot of time to set up a show. It takes a

concentrated effort that demands giving yourself totally to the show. There can be no time for anything else . . . or anyone else." She said the last words in almost a whisper.

Heather heard Reid's chair scrape the floor as he stood up. Then she sensed him standing only inches from her. She felt the warmth of his breath as it brushed across her cheek. "Don't wait too long. Don't waste what you have," he said.

Heather did not trust herself to move or speak with him that close to her. She stood stiffly, her breathing shallow, until she heard him turn and start away.

"I'll go take care of some paperwork and leave you alone," Reid said from the doorway.

Heather could only nod at him. Her head spun and her thoughts were even more confused than before Reid had come into the office. Although she had listened intently to what he said about the ranch, there had been one corner of her mind that kept returning to his barely checked anger that had flared when she had called herself stupid. After an initial moment of fright at his unexpected response to her self-pity, Heather had realized he would not have been so angered, would not have reacted so strongly, if he did not— *No!* She refused to allow the word to enter her thoughts. *Wait,* she told herself. *Be patient until he's ready.*

Polaris laid his head on Heather's lap at the same instant that she heard the muffled sound of Reid moving about in his office. After several seconds she guessed he had seated himself at his desk and begun his work.

Would she see him tonight, she wondered as she stood and patted her thigh, Polaris's signal to heel. "Come on, boy, let's take a nice long walk."

Chapter Thirteen

*H*eather sat on her couch, aware that midnight had come and gone. She was listening to the night sounds that entered through the open living room windows. Insects and one old owl that Heather had been listening to for years were the only sounds that broke the stillness.

It was very different from just a few hours ago, when the ranch had been alive with the returning cowboys. The men's shouting, bragging, and general joviality had helped to lift her from the mild depression that had been holding her in its grip.

Now, sitting on the couch in the same clothing she had put on after taking a shower before dinner, Heather wondered if she should undress and go to bed or if she dared to visit Reid.

As she stood smoothing her skirt and fluffing her shoulder-length hair, she realized she had no choice. If she did go to bed, she would not be able to sleep. She had to talk with Reid.

Walking slowly to the front door, Heather wondered if Reid liked blue. The wide skirt she wore was a color that Emma had once told her matched her eyes. Her top was an off-white peasant blouse that was light and comfortable with flaring sleeves ending at her wrists and a scoop neck that showed just the barest hint of her breasts. Heather knew the skirt and blouse accentuated the slimness of her waist. It was also the perfect outfit to lounge around in—not too dressy or provocative.

Heather paused for a moment at the door, wondering if she had subconsciously planned to see Reid tonight and dressed for it. Shrugging the thought away, she opened the front door.

Descending the three wooden steps, Heather turned toward the small house that Reid Hunter now called home. Before she had taken five steps, Polaris came to her side. She scratched the large dog under one ear without breaking her stride.

Polaris must have sensed where Heather was headed because he stopped her just before Reid's steps and barked once. "Sshh," Heather said quickly. "Run," she added. Polaris stayed for a moment, and again Heather sensed the protectiveness that seemed to emanate from the dog. "Go," she said again in a low voice. Again he disobeyed her as he lay down at the foot of the steps.

"Okay, be stubborn!" she said as she stepped over the large dog and onto the first step.

It was easier this time, Heather thought as she knocked on Reid's door. The door opened quickly and she stepped inside.

"You knew?" she asked.

"I hoped," Reid replied. Heather caught her breath at his words and reached out her hand. His hand covered hers quickly and she felt the familiar warmth of his skin. Slowly, she brought his hand to her lips and tasted its back.

Before she was aware of what was happening, she was enfolded in his arms. Her breasts were flattened against his chest and her breathing was strained before his lips touched hers. When they did, the fires that had burst forth so wildly last night returned, blazing even stronger. She felt like the molten metal she would be using to cast Reid's likeness and knew that what she had thought before was true—she had no choice, she had to be here with him.

Her hands ran along Reid's beautifully muscled back, feeling the texture of his skin through the shirt he wore. The heat from his loins burned through the thickness of his jeans, and tremors from his thighs seemed to run the length of her own body. And then he pulled away. He held her at arm's length and Heather instinctively knew he was looking deeply into her eyes.

"We have to talk," Reid said. Heather heard him try to control his breathing as he waited for her words. She sensed how affected he was by the kiss and how hard it had been for him to stop.

"We talked last night. I know what you want to say."

"It's more than that," Reid began.

"There's only one thing I want to hear," she said, cutting him off. She held her breath, shocked at the suddenness of the words she had not intended to speak. From the sound of his breathing, Heather also knew he understood.

Reid stood there looking at her, knowing that if he denied it, knowing that if he did not speak, that nothing would change. The way he felt would have no affect on his words. It would be easier to deny his feelings, to refuse to acknowledge the inevitable. Slowly, tasting the dryness of his mouth, he stepped closer to her and put his hands on her shoulders. He looked down, seeing her face and the tense lines that pulled at the corners of her mouth. He had learned in the months of working on the ranch to look at Heather's mouth. Like most people's eyes, the set of Heather's softly curved lips was an indication of her inner thoughts.

"Heather, you are the most beautiful, most desirable woman I have ever touched or made love to. Whenever I look at you, I want you. I want to hold you and make love to you. But we can't," he said in a hoarse voice. "Go now! Leave!"

"No!" Heather stood taller as she defied him, drawing on her inner strength and resolve. "I told you everything was settled. You don't have to say anything. But if you do, say what you feel, not what you think you have to."

"Damn it, Heather! Do you think I'm made of the same clay you work with every day? Do you think that I have no emotions, that I can live easily, making love to you at night and waking up in the morning to an empty bed? Do you think it's easy to speak about, to tell you how I feel and know it can only be said in the dead of the night so no one can hear?" Reid whispered, unable to control the tightness in his voice.

"No, Reid, it's not easy," Heather said, reeling under the assault of his words, the words of longing, passion, and denial. She was stung as much by the fierceness of his reply as by the pressure of his fingers digging harshly into the skin of her shoulders. "I . . . I'll go," she said, fighting back the tears that threatened to spill. She eased from his grip and turned. Silence filled her ears as she walked the few steps to the door. When her hand was on the knob, she wanted to turn back, to tell him to pretend she had not spoken. But she would not do that to him.

Reid watched her go to the door and open it. A darkness invaded his mind and he deliberately closed his eyes. *Let her go,* he told himself.

Turning the doorknob was torture to Heather. An eternity of time passed as her hand moved slowly. Then the door was opening.

"I love you," came Reid's voice. Heather froze. The door was half open. She wasn't sure whether he had said it or it had been a trick of her mind, born of a desperate need.

"Don't pretend you didn't hear me! I said I love you. Now close the damn door and turn around!"

Heather closed the door and turned, unheeding of the tears that streamed down her face. She did not hear him move, but the fiery trail his fingers made as they wiped her tears told her he was with her.

Then she was in his arms, pressing against the hardness that was his body, drawing in the heat he radiated. Her lips hungrily sought and found his. And as their tongues met, their hands pulled each other so tightly that Heather grew dizzy. A moment later they parted, but this time Reid kept silent as he walked with her toward his bedroom.

Heather understood that they had just passed into a different level of their relationship. The rules would be the same, but she knew they would hide less from each other and be able to share things that could not have existed without his admission. True, they would still be limited to their private world, but they could now make this world broader for themselves.

The dam burst within him when Reid finally admitted his love. He was furious with himself for speaking of it, for allowing himself the weakness that would ultimately cause Heather pain.

That was why he had refused himself any involvements during the last ten years. That was why, when he felt the need of a woman's company, he had always gone to the places where he would find a woman for the night, and when he awoke the next day, he knew he would never see her again. But this morning, when he had awakened alone, the loss he'd felt had started the destruction of his resolve. Watching Heather at the door had been the final point. He loved her, and because he did, he was condemning her to a life of hiding.

Without being aware of it, he had led Heather into his bedroom. He paused to look at her. Her tears had stopped and the corners of her mouth were relaxed. She was beautiful, he thought as the desire that had flamed through him when they had kissed earlier began to rise anew. He wanted, and needed, to make love to her.

Reid lowered his mouth to hers and tasted her lips again. His mind ceased to function and he became lost in her. The hunger he had denied himself for so long burst forth and claimed them both.

Heather felt his mouth on hers and felt his hands again on her shoulders as he pulled her against him. Then they were moving again, and in a haze that blurred her mind's perception, they undressed and fell onto the soft down quilt.

With every touch on her skin Heather felt new sensations burst free. His hands, although calloused from years of ranch work, moved with a gentleness that told her even more of his love for her. With every movement he made Heather became more aware of her feelings for Reid. His lips sought new paths on her body, causing her to twist and turn as she held him against her. His lips were everywhere that his hands had been, teasing, soothing, pulling, and giving until she could stand no more and wove her fingers into his hair. She pulled him to her, kissing him deeply until finally they joined together, sealing the love they had spoken of.

This time was different from before as she fought to maintain an edge on reality while Reid carried her again to the highest reaches of the heavens. But try as she might, all her senses centered on her man, the touch, the sound, the feel, and the aura of Reid Hunter as he made love to her. Time after time, Heather was lifted to a new sense of freedom that was made possible only within Reid's arms.

Reid held Heather close to him, losing himself within the softness of her skin and the warmth of her femininity. His hands roamed her body, even as he made love to her, seeking to learn everything he could. He held his eyes closed, as he had not done last night, letting his other senses become aware of the woman under him. His mouth was in her hair and he smelled the very essence of her. His hands ran along her sides, feeling her silkiness until he could no longer guide himself. Turning the control of his mind over to his senses, Reid moved with her, joining her completely, giving himself to her as he had never before done with another.

Together they reached a shared plateau that held only themselves. Together, on the velvet softness of what they had created between them, they held each other until sleep stole them away.

"No! No! Bastards!" Heather was pulled from the depths of her sleep by the words Reid was shouting. She felt herself tremble at the emotions that his ragged breathing conveyed. Unnamed horrors filled her mind as she brought herself to full awareness, pushing aside the memory of their lovemaking as her hand went to his face.

Reid was bathed in icy sweat; his head jerked from side to side as he spoke. Slowly, carefully, Heather pressed herself against his large body, using her hands to soothe and draw him from his nightmare.

After several agonizing seconds, Reid's head stopped moving and his breathing returned to normal. "I'm okay," he whispered.

"Is it always this bad?" she asked, remembering a conversation they had had a few days ago about his dreams.

"Always."

"Will you tell me about it?" Heather bit her lip after she asked the question. She should not have, but she had to. It seemed that everything she thought or did concerning Reid Hunter had other ramifications that she had not taken into consideration. Reid's body stiffened and she felt the tension throbbing within him as if it were a tangible item and understood another battle was being fought within his mind.

"You don't have to," she added in a whisper. Suddenly she felt him relax and he took her hand in his. She enjoyed the gentle pressure he exerted and relief flooded her mind.

Reid held her hand, his mind again in turmoil as it always was after one of his dreams. Only sheer willpower had enabled him to yield, to make his body relax. Holding Heather's smaller hand in his, he wondered if he could tell her what had happened. He also wondered if she would be able to handle what he had done and still feel the same way toward him.

"Reid?" came Heather's whisper.

"It was a long time ago," he said as he tried to make his decision. "A long time ago in another country—another world." Fully conscious of what he was doing and knowing the possible consequences, Reid began to speak.

He told her of that fateful patrol, of the arrogant captain who would not listen to the more experienced men. He felt the tension build in her body as he held her closer to his side, conscious of the soft feel of her naked skin against his. But there was also reassurance in her hand as it continually brushed soothingly through his hair.

When he reached the point when the patrol was in the village, he paused for a moment, aware of the cold sweat that again bathed his body. Heather had not moved and he knew she could feel it also.

His words evoked the pictures of what had happened as he spoke of it aloud for the first time since returning from overseas. The words flowed smoothly until he finally had to admit the truth of what had happened there. He told Heather in clinical detail what he had done. When he was finished, he looked at her and waited.

"It wasn't your fault," Heather said, waiting for a long time after Reid had finished before speaking. Her mind had been numbed by his story. The horror he had described had made her feel as sick as he had been in Vietnam. But over the years she had heard many stories, especially in school, when the war was ending. And Heather also knew the type of man Reid Hunter was, and that he was not a killer. His curse was in the fact that he was an idealist.

"They shot at you and you didn't know who it was until afterward. Reid, you never even fired a shot. You didn't kill them!"

"I know that, but my men were my responsibility. It's the same as if I fired, too," Reid said as he took a deep breath. "But that doesn't bring back two children and a woman from the dead. The little boy who shot Trigent didn't know what he was doing. Their village had been attacked time and time again by both the Cong and the Americans. The boy was just reacting. He was too young to understand. Heather, he was younger than Gregg Farley!"

"And that's why you're punishing yourself?" Heather asked as she pulled herself even closer to him, trying to comfort him with her body as much as her words. "It wasn't your fault. You and your men were trained to have an instinctive response to danger, not to analyze it first. It's been a long time. You can't carry your guilt forever."

"I can't shed it like a snakeskin either. I've been trying to make up for it ever since. The children were the victims of this war, and I was part of the war."

"That's what the Foundation is all about, isn't it? That's why you were able to arrange for the loan and the camp," Heather stated, thinking she understood Reid's role better now. "But you can't spend the rest of your life making up for what you could not have prevented."

"I haven't had much choice," he said. Then Reid saw another truth. Heather had not run from him, had not turned away in disgust when he'd told his story. In actuality, it had been just the opposite. She had come closer to him.

"Reid, what happened to you was a . . . a terrible but unpreventable accident. That doesn't make it right, but neither does running away from your own life give those children back their lives."

"I haven't been running away from what happened

to me in the war," Reid told her, feeling the sting of truth in her words. "I've learned to live with that. Now, I need you to kiss me." Heather felt tears well up in her eyes from his request. She moved along his length until her lips were on his. When she tasted the saltiness of his mouth, she could no longer restrain herself and again her tears flowed freely. Together they held each other until the fierceness of their emotions subsided.

"I love you, Reid, for who you are. Remember that, and never doubt it," she said.

Reid heard her words and pressed her tightly against him. He kissed her, tasting the woman that she was, and again heat flowed between them.

Heather felt and tried to absorb all his pain and anguish within her as she kissed him. She realized now why he had tried to avoid their love. No longer would she wonder about him. She would just love him, on his terms.

Once again they came together, gently and tenderly, drawing comfort and giving each other love in the early hours before the dawn.

Chapter Fourteen

With the July sun bathing her in its midday warmth and the grass soft beneath her, Heather lay near the edge of the pond. As the sensitive fingers of one hand absently stroked the sleeping shepherd lying next to her, the fingers of her other hand rambled through the grass, pausing to feel the texture of each individual blade before moving on to the next. This grass was special; it had been planted by her mother, just after her father had dug and filled the man-made pond, and was different from all other varieties found on the ranch. The grass's smooth surface combined with the coarser, almost sawlike edges was a tactile massage Heather could appreciate. A blade of grass, she thought, was so fragile yet so tough. Grass gave life to barren land, gave strength to grazing animals, and gave comfort to feet that walked upon it.

For a ranch, grassy plains, rolling plateaus, and rich

valleys were its lifeblood, whether they be buffalo grass, Indian rice grass, sagebrush, or any of the other multitudes of vegetation found in Nevada. Ranching demanded much from those who would reap its benefits, and those benefits, too, were like the grass— smooth, with rough edges. You had to be strong to live, fight, and succeed. And you needed strong people to help you, people who were like the blades of grass she held in her fingers—strong, sharp, but at the same time loving, gentle, and giving.

Like Reid. The name rolled thunderously within the pathways of her mind. Like Reid—the smoothness of his skin and the rippling of the hard muscles that lay just beneath the surface, the calloused hands that could grasp a rope and make it do whatever he willed, and the gentleness of those hands as they had roamed the contours of her body. Like Reid—soft, hard, firm, yielding, intractable. And like the single blade of grass she suddenly broke off, there was so much more beneath the surface.

In the days and nights that flowed into weeks following that fateful weekend of their discovery of love, Heather had begun to live on a tightrope that balanced between two worlds. She had the day-to-day world of the Strand Ranch and the nighttime world of her love. She worked, spoke, and interacted with Reid in her role as owner, with him as foreman. At night, when the ranch slept, she loved and was loved. After those first nights of lovemaking, of discovering each other, of admissions and long-buried truths, they began to become a couple.

Heather could almost feel Reid next to her as her fingers continued to explore the grass. Night was the time she truly came to life. The learning about each other, the hours spent talking and then falling asleep in his arms, far exceeded the nights spent in passion. But with each waking Heather had felt renewed. Just being with him, talking, holding, touching—those things had become so vital. Not even those lonely walks home, before Reid and the ranch woke, were able to diminish the strength of her feelings.

And now, although it was not five months since she'd hired Reid, the ranch was beginning to grow again. The money from the loan had already been used beneficially.

Reid had told her in full detail of the plans that he'd drawn up for the possible cattle-ranching operation. Accompanied by Heather and Tom Farley, Reid had gone to talk with one of the smaller local provisioners about supplying him with prime-grade beef at a low but fair price under the stipulation that the meat would be sold only in local markets, to the smaller, independent businesses rather than to the larger resorts, whose inflated prices were meant for the tourists. This way they would not be in competition with the larger ranchers who sold for a higher margin of profit and expected their beef to go to the major market for top dollar. The amount of cattle the Strand Ranch would be selling would not make a noticeable difference to the larger ranchers but would help to stabilize the ranch financially. The distributor had seemed both impressed and agreeable to their ideas.

And just last week, Heather thought, the first of the new breeding studs had arrived. The stallion was a Thoroughbred/Morgan mix who Reid was positive would sire the type of foal that would grow into a strong and tough range horse, a similar breed to the horses that the Strand Ranch had become known for in the past. Heather also realized that the stud signaled the beginning of the return of the Strand Ranch to the position it had held for many years.

Yes, she thought, everything was turning out well. The ranch was on the upswing, thanks to Reid's capable guidance. The problems that had plagued Heather and the ranch were disappearing one by one—all except her newest problem.

Heather pulled out another blade of grass and passed it back and forth across her lips. The tickling sensation felt good, but she could not shake the ugly thought that had arisen. Her problem, she admitted, was herself.

It had been a small thought at first, hidden in one of the many compartments of her mind. She had tried to keep it closed off from herself, but the harder she tried, the more urgent the problem became. Heather recognized the fact that she was questioning the very basis of her relationship with Reid.

In the beginning she had accepted the rules that governed them. But her mind would not let it stay there. Something told her that it was more than the antiquated cowboy creed that governed their relationship. She knew, too, that it was more than just his haunting Vietnamese past that held him back. But just what it was she couldn't figure out.

There were too many small items that, when put together, did not add up. Reid's way of always finding the right thing to say and his ability to articulate above the level of his background had started to bother her. His artfulness in building stone walls that deflected the most direct and penetrating personal questions made her wonder what he was really hiding from.

There was something stopping Reid Hunter from acknowledging his love for her openly, and it was more than his being her foreman. Heather also realized that not since the time when he'd told her to leave and her hand was on the doorknob and he had said I love you had he repeated it.

Heather tensed. The one thing she tried to avoid came roaring into her mind; her throat tightened painfully and she felt moisture rise into her eyes. *I was the one who forced everything*, she reminded herself. *I went after Reid. I pushed myself on him at every opportunity. My feelings must have been more than obvious in everything I did. Emma saw it plainly, and Reid must have thought he had no choice.*

Then Heather's tortured thoughts told her something else, something that made her cringe inside. She remembered Reid telling her how desirable she was, how beautiful she was. *But am I? Was he only telling me what I wanted to hear? How do I know if I'm desirable, if I'm really beautiful? I don't. I can't. I can only believe what I'm told.*

Was Reid using her? Another memory came, one that she was ashamed of. She had been walking the other night and had passed Reid's house. She had heard Reid and Tom talking loudly, arguing. She had stopped, knowing she shouldn't, and listened. She had been able to hear some of the words, but not all. Again she replayed the conversation in her mind.

"Why'd you lie," Tom had asked. Heather had stiffened at the harshness of Tom's voice.

"Lie?" she had heard Reid reply.

" 'Bout who you . . ." Heather had not heard the last word and had strained harder.

"How'd you find out?" Reid had said, and she had felt her stomach knot.

"I met someone who works at the . . . We talked for a while. Seems he knew you a long time. . . ." Tom had said, but again, Heather had missed some of the words.

"Higgins?" had come Reid's response.

"Yes. Reid, I like you. I don't understand what you're doing, but I can't believe you're working this hard for nothing. I just want to know one thing," Tom had said.

Heather had heard only silence for a few moments, and then she had heard Tom speak again. "Are you doing this for . . ."

Again, Heather had missed the word. Her heart was telling her to leave, not to listen to more, but her mind had fought and won. She had to hear it out.

"Higgins has a big mouth," Reid had replied, his voice stronger and filled with more confidence. "I'm not here for any other reason than for the job I took. I'm here to get this place back on its feet. My family has nothing to do with this. They don't know where I am!" Reid had finished. These new words had Heather's mind spinning. ". . . here to do a job. My family has nothing to do with this." *My family!* The words had kept repeating endlessly in her mind as she stood there in the night.

"I want to believe that," Tom had said.

"Believe it. It's the truth," Reid had replied.

"I think it is. Reid, as I said before, I like you. I won't say anything 'bout this," Heather heard Tom promise.

About what? her mind had screamed. Hearing the voices grow louder, Heather started to walk away. Her mind had been in shock and she had spent the night alone, trying to comprehend what had happened. Her only point of reference was Tom Farley, who had told Reid he trusted him. Unless she told Tom about herself and Reid, she too had to trust him. So she had pushed the conversation she had overheard to the back of her mind, hoping her own dark thoughts would stay there.

But the thoughts had returned. What family did Reid have? There had been no mention on his resume of family, no mention of a wife. Had he done that purposely? Was he married? Was that why he wanted their love hidden? Had she let herself become a plaything for her foreman. *No!* her heart cried. Heather knew that it was something else. Not knowing how, she knew he was not married. But the mystery remained lodged within her mind, and she knew she would have to find out.

Heather could no longer be satisfied with a hidden, nighttime love that left with the arrival of the sun.

Polaris raised his head quickly, dislodging Heather's hand in the process and bringing her thoughts back to the grass she was lying on. A low *woof* escaped Polaris's throat and she felt the breeze from his wagging tail as he stood.

Heather sat up as she heard her name called out. "Miss Heather," Gregg Farley said, catching his breath as he stopped running. "Miss Emma sent me to fetch you."

"It must be mighty important for you to be so out of breath," she said to him as she willed her troubled thoughts away and smiled at the boy.

"I don't know if it is, but I've been lookin' everywhere for you. This was my last try 'fore I gave up."

"I told Emma I'd be here," Heather said, puzzled as to why Emma hadn't told Gregg.

"She said so, but when I came by before I didn't see you. I didn't 'spect you to be lyin' down."

"Don't you ever lie in the grass?" Heather asked as she stood, stretched, and began to walk.

"Yes'm. But I never seen you lie in it before."

"Saw," she corrected.

"I never saw you lyin' down on the grass before,"

Gregg repeated, carefully choosing the right words. At the office door Gregg said good-bye to Heather, returning to his school friend, who was visiting him for the day.

Heather stepped into the air-conditioned coolness of Emma's office and shivered at the instant change of temperature.

"You called?" Heather said as she shivered again. "Are you trying to freeze to death?" she asked the older woman.

"It's barely comfortable in here, and, no, I didn't call. I sent a messenger for you. If I had called, I would have frightened your new stallion half to death."

"Emma!" Heather drawled out her friend's name in exasperation.

"Take it easy. I have some papers for you to sign, and I have to get to the bank before it closes."

"Which ones?"

"The ones that are on your desk—the license applications for the camp," Emma reminded her. Heather remembered and smiled as she went into her office with Emma trailing behind. She stopped at the front of her desk and held out her hand for a pen. Emma handed her the pen, then guided her hand to the spot. Heather signed the three copies and put the pen down with a flourish.

"Ta-ta," she said as she stood up again.

"Now, my dear, if you'll excuse me, I'm off to town." Heather smiled and nodded. She heard Emma open the door and then pause as the echo of a car door being closed reached her ears. "I wonder who that could be?" Emma said, and Heather heard her turn and walk to the window. "Expecting any visitors?" she asked Heather.

"No. What does he look like?"

"Tall and thin, with long dark hair about waist length."

"I take it it's a woman, not a man."

"So does Tom Farley. A very pretty one. His mouth just fell wide open. Whew—he made a good recovery."

"Emma, what's going on?" Heather asked.

"We'll soon find out. Tom and the lady are headed this way. Have a nice afternoon. Think about what we've discussed. I'll see you about four," Emma said as she left the office, quietly closing the door behind her very confused boss.

Heather stood between the door and the desk, smiling at Emma's last words. The outer office door closed loudly and she heard Emma greet Tom, but missed the low-voiced introductions. Taking a deep breath, Heather stood and went to the door. Her hand was on the knob when she heard the static of the CB fill the air. She paused then, for some unknown reason.

Tom's voice, loud as was his habit when he used the radio, carried clearly through the closed door. "Rover One, come in," he said. Heather opened the door slightly, when she heard him calling Reid.

"Rover One," came the voice.

"Reid, you've got a visitor. When are you heading back?" Tom asked. Heather tensed as she heard Tom's question, realizing the visitor was for Reid. A strange sensation akin to anger began to creep into Heather's mind as she listened intently.

"I'm not expecting anyone, but I'm already on the way back. Who is it?" Reid asked.

"One of the two prettiest sights I've seen on this ranch in a long time," Tom said. Heather felt another surge of anger spread throughout her body, and because of it failed to notice the different way that Tom Farley sounded.

"You want to run that by me again?" Reid request-ed. Heather heard the woman take two steps and then heard her voice.

"You always were the slow one," she said.

"Gwen?" Heather heard the doubt that filled Reid's voice. "What the hell . . ." Reid said, cutting himself off in midsentence. "I'll be there in ten minutes. Rover One, out."

Suddenly Heather understood what was happening to her. She was jealous! Jealous of the way Reid sounded, jealous of this woman she did not know, and feeling again the knot of tension in her stomach. Was this the family that Reid and Tom had talked about? Heather closed the door quietly and went to her chair. She sat for a few minutes, and when her mind had calmed, she stood. As she did, she heard a knock on her door.

"Heather," Tom called. Heather went to the door and opened it, a feeling of dread holding her in thrall.

"Yes, Tom?"

"There's someone here I'd like you to meet," he said, taking her arm and guiding her into the main office. "Heather Strand, I'd like you to meet Gwen Hunter, Reid's sister." A wave of relief flooded through her at Tom's words.

"A pleasure, Miss Strand," Gwen said. Heath-er heard the woman take several steps toward her and she moved in the direction of Gwen Hunter's voice. She held out her hand and it was grasped by Gwen. She liked the feeling of the handshake. It was cool, firm, and decisive.

"Call me Heather. Glad to meet you," she said truthfully as she released the other woman's hand.

"I hope you don't mind my coming here so unexpect-edly?"

"It's no problem, Gwen, although I think I heard a bit of shock in your brother's voice."

"He'll get over it . . . I hope," Gwen finished. "Please, don't let me stop you from your work. I'll just wait here for Reid. Mr. Farley, thank you for your help."

"You're welcome," Tom said. A quiet moment passed before Tom spoke again. "I guess I'd better get back to work. I hope I'll see you later, Miss Gwen."

"I hope so too," she replied. "That's if Reid doesn't break my neck."

"Don't you worry about him. He wouldn't do that. Your neck's too pretty." Heather couldn't believe her ears. But before she could say a word, the office door closed and Tom was gone.

"My goodness, you must be something. I've never heard Tom say anything like that."

"He is cute, though, isn't he?" Gwen said in a faraway voice.

"I've never heard Tom called cute either," Heather replied.

"Oh, didn't you see the way he blushed just before he left?" Gwen asked.

"No, I'm afraid I didn't," Heather said lightly. Suddenly she sensed Gwen peering at her and Heather knew Gwen hadn't realized until then that she was blind. "Why don't you sit and relax. I'm sure Reid will be here any moment."

"Thank you again," Gwen said. Heather noted no change in Gwen's voice and was surprised. Usually when somebody discovered she was blind they sounded different, more hesitant, as if trying to choose the correct words to express their sorrow. "I bet it hasn't been easy, running this place," Gwen added.

"Excuse me?"

"Being a woman, I mean. I grew up on a ranch. Women aren't exactly a cowboy's idea of a boss."

"You can say that again," Heather joked as Gwen's words brought a rush of warmth to her and a feeling of instant kinship with her.

The sound of the Land-Rover pulling to a stop ended any further conversation. The hard slam of the vehicle's door told both women about Reid's mood when he walked into the office. But before he could greet his sister, Heather spoke up.

"Reid, I've work to do in the studio. When you leave here, would you call me? Emma won't be back until later." Without waiting for a reply Heather turned to Gwen. "It was a pleasure meeting you. I hope you'll be around for a few days."

"Thank you. You're very kind," Gwen said softly. Heather smiled at Gwen and then left for her studio. She had started work on a new piece two days ago but was having trouble transferring her idea to the clay. She wanted to try again today, and Reid's being in the office freed her for a little while.

Walking to her studio, Heather's thoughts were on her instant liking of Gwen Hunter and on Tom Farley's strange reaction to Reid's sister.

Chapter Fifteen

The slanting sun was just below the window of Reid's kitchen, where he and Gwen now sat. When they had been left alone in the office, Gwen had begun to tell him why she'd come, but Reid had stopped her. He'd told her he wanted more privacy than the office offered. He'd pointed out his house to her, sending her there to put her things away and wait for him. Then, conscious of her presence on the ranch, Reid had concentrated on paperwork until Emma returned.

Reid gazed warily across the length of the small white Formica table as he tried to field Gwen's questions. She had always been intuitive, always able to hear the words Reid left unsaid. He had been hesitant in asking her not to mention anything about Broadlands or their past when anyone from the Strand Ranch was near. She had raised one dark eyebrow in question as they sipped their coffee, watching each other.

"Have I ever done anything like that before? We

agreed a long time ago that no one would know about your past. Why are you reminding me?" Gwen asked.

"You've never before just shown up at a place I work. I wasn't prepared."

"There's more to it," Gwen stated knowingly.

"A lot more," Reid agreed with a flash of white teeth and a flinty-eyed stare that said he wouldn't go any further.

"You're different somehow. I sensed it the minute I saw you. You're more . . . relaxed," Gwen said after a second's hesitation. Gwen's eyes, as hazel as her brother's, washed across his face contemplatively. "The dreams?" Reid nodded.

"I still have them, but they're fading. They're not as intense anymore, not since—" Reid bit off the last word, suddenly aware he was saying too much.

Reid watched his sister's eyes plead silently for him to go on. When she realized he wasn't going to, she shrugged. "Whatever," she said.

"Why did you come after I told you I wouldn't go back?"

"Why did you come when I called for your help six years ago?" Gwen answered his question with one of her own.

"Because you needed me."

"Patrick needs you now."

"Patrick can go to hell!"

"Along with Broadlands?" Gwen snapped the question suddenly. "My God, Reid, don't you think I know what Pat is? Don't you think I know what he's done to you—and to me? But that's not the issue. Our entire past is about to disappear."

"I thought you didn't know what was happening at Broadlands."

"When I spoke to you, I didn't. Chet was mad at Pat,

but his loyalty was still there and he wouldn't say anything, so I started to check on what was happening." Gwen paused and stood, drawing herself up to her full five-foot-eleven-inch height. She smiled sadly down at Reid before she went to the stove. She took the coffeepot and brought it back to the table. "Coffee?" At Reid's patient nod Gwen filled both cups and set the pot on the table.

"After I spoke to you, I decided to dig into it and find out what was happening." Gwen took a sip of coffee and stared at her brother for a long moment before continuing. "The problem began shortly after you left. I should have seen it then, but I didn't. Pat was crazy. I guess he needed to prove that he could do everything on the ranch without you. Broadlands was doing fine— at least, when I left. But in the last few years things haven't gone well for him.

"He overstocked when the new FDA procedures went into effect. He wanted to build up prime stock and then make a big-profit sale. Only it didn't work out. There was an epidemic of hoof and mouth two years ago."

"I didn't hear a thing about it," Reid interrupted.

"It was contained. Only three ranches in Albuquerque were affected. Broadlands was hit the worst. Two-thirds of the herd was infected—the government ordered the rest destroyed for protection."

Reid paled. The words his sister spoke were the fear of any rancher. He knew without asking what the losses to Broadlands were.

"Pat used every penny he had in the bank to buy new stock and he almost pulled it off," Gwen said. Reid held his sister's eyes with his own as he nodded slowly.

"The market fell heavily last year," he finished for her.

Gwen nodded. "He had to sell. He had no choice. He lost again."

"I can't believe it," Reid whispered.

"Pat sold five thousand acres of land three months ago. That's what he and Chet fought over."

"He what?" Reid's question exploded as the back of his hand slammed into his coffee cup, sending it flying across the kitchen.

"He sold off five thousand acres of Papa's land, our land."

"He had no right," Reid whispered, still feeling the shock of Gwen's words.

"He had every right. We gave it to him. We both signed the power of attorneys giving him full charge."

"Not to sell the land," Reid defended.

"To do anything he wants. But that's not the real problem. The real problem is why I'm here now."

"What's the real problem?" Reid demanded, his voice harsh with emotion.

"Pat needs help. He needs you to help him. I think he's going to sell off more land," Gwen said quickly, taking a rasping breath before speaking again. "When I was checking on this, I spoke to Mr. Samuels at the bank. He told me he felt odd about setting up the paperwork."

"He should. Broadlands has supported that bank for over fifty years. Gwen, did you talk to Pat?"

"He told me that once I left I had no say in what he did."

"He's right, but he's wrong," Reid told her, a sudden smile on his face.

"He must be hurting very badly," Gwen ventured.

"But not bad enough to break down and call us," Reid replied, unable to hide the acid that filled his voice.

"For what?" Gwen asked, puzzled.

Reid ignored Gwen's question for a moment as he chased the idea that had jumped into his head.

"Reid?" Gwen called in a low voice. Reid gazed at her, his mind slowing as the idea fell into place. "Please come back with me. We'll talk to Pat. He'll have to face us and work it out."

"No."

"Can't you forget what's happened? He won't tell you, but he needs you . . . us!" Gwen said, desperation making her voice strong.

"I know," Reid said softly. But not even the relief that was evident on Gwen's face could stop the sudden flow of anger his thoughts had brought on. "I'll go, not you."

"Both of us."

"He won't be able to handle that. He can't face both of us and bare his weakness. I'll go, not you," Reid repeated, holding his sister's eyes with a riveting stare. He waited, unbending, until she nodded her head in agreement.

"You two are so different, yet so alike," she said.

"I have some work to finish tomorrow. I'll fly to Albuquerque tomorrow night," Reid said as he stood and stretched. "There're some spare sheets in the closet. You, little sister, can make up the couch for yourself. I think I've given up enough for one night."

"Reid, thank you," Gwen said. Reid saw her moisture-laden eyes and walked over to her, pulled her to her feet, and hugged her tightly.

"I'm going for a walk. I'll be back in a little while."

Heather sat on her front steps, breathing in the cool night air. The summer had not turned as hot as she had anticipated, and there hadn't been another really warm night since the night she'd gone swimming in the pond. But she would rather have the cool mountain breezes each night than the hot and arid air that covered so much of the state in summer.

Nearby, blending with yet distinct from the night sounds, Heather heard Polaris's paws as he ran across the ground. He, too, was enjoying this evening. She heard him stop suddenly, and his low but friendly growl of recognition carried to her ears. Someone he had recognized was outside. Heather wondered if it was Reid.

With the arrival of Reid's sister Heather knew she would probably not see him tonight. But that did not stop her desires. A quick smile appeared on her face as she recalled Tom's vivid description of Gwen Hunter earlier that evening. Gwen Hunter had found a new admirer today; Tom's voice had held ample proof of that.

"She sure is pretty," Tom had said, standing behind Heather in the studio. "I've never seen a woman that tall who looked so good and walked so smoothly. You know, her eyes are the same color as Reid's, but with just a bit more green in them. Her face has character—it's not just pretty, but it's got . . . I don't know, but when she smiles, all those laugh lines around her eyes crinkle up and it sure looks good."

"What's her neck like?" Heather had asked.

"Her neck? I . . . er . . ." Tom had stuttered.

"You're the one who said it was too nice to break," Heather reminded him. She heard him shuffle his feet for a moment before he spoke.

"To tell you the truth, Heather, that was just a figure of speech. She was wearing a lacy shirt with a high collar. I didn't really see her neck."

Heather chuckled softly at the memory. Then she started to wonder what might happen if Gwen stayed at the ranch for a few days. She sobered instantly. What would happen between her and Reid if Gwen stayed for a while? Could anything more, or less, happen?

"Heather?" Reid's voice called. For just a moment she thought she was imagining it, until she felt Polaris sit at her feet and Reid sit next to her.

"Good evening," she said softly.

"I need to speak with you for a few minutes."

"Here?"

"This is fine, or we could walk."

"I'd like that," she said as she stood. Her heart screamed for him to take her into his arms. They walked silently in the direction of the corral. Heather, striding between Reid and Polaris, felt tension radiating from Reid as she waited for him to begin. When they were close to the corral, Heather felt the now familiar sensation of electricity as Reid's hand took hers and pressed it gently.

"I've got some family problems. I'll have to leave for a few days," he told her.

"I'm sorry," Heather said, ineffectually covering the leaping of her heart.

"It shouldn't take more than a couple of days, and Tom can handle everything until I get back. Four days at the most," he added.

There were a million questions she wanted to ask, but she was still reluctant to break the unspoken rules they had established, even after her afternoon of introspection.

"I'll miss you," Heather whispered, struggling amid the sudden surge of emotions the words brought to her.

"Heather, I . . ." Reid began as he looked at her,

framed by moonlight. He understood everything she had not said and watched as she proudly held her head high. "I'll miss you, too."

"Do you love me, Reid?" Before he could answer Heather moved against him, uncaring of any eyes that might be on them, disregarding for once the rules that had been established, not caring if he were to draw away. But this time Reid didn't. His lips covered hers and she felt herself melt into his arms. Warmth spread throughout her body and mind. After a long, torturous minute, Heather pulled back, turning away as her hand sought and found his. As suddenly as her need to kiss him had come, another need had followed. She needed to talk to him—not about their love, but about herself. She had spent many hours thinking about this.

"Do you like my sculptures?" she asked, again not allowing him to answer her first question.

"Yes," he said truthfully.

"You know, you've really changed the ranch. You've made a big difference here."

"Not that big, not yet. There's lots more to do."

"But it's started. You've also made something else possible. My retirement."

"Retirement?" Reid echoed.

"I learned something today. It's you who runs the ranch—you, Tom, and Emma. All I do is say yes when you ask something and put my signature on the line when I'm told to sign. I'm useless. This ranch is too small for a good foreman and a working owner. I guess that's why my father never had a strong foreman." Heather paused for a breath before she went on, and when she did, Reid saw a change on her face. "I'm useless as a rancher. I've been thinking about becoming a real artist—not just someone who plays with clay."

"You *are* a *real* artist. You're one of the best I've ever seen!" Reid stated. "I'm glad to hear that you're going to work on your art."

"Thank you, but I'm just beginning. It takes a lot of work and time to develop a style and become recognized. In order to do that, I've got to work on a collection for a show. It will involve a lot of time, and I just wanted to make sure . . ." Heather stopped, aware she did not know precisely what she wanted to say. Cursing her foolishness, she spoke again. "What I mean is that, when I'm ready, when it's time for me to have a showing, I'll have to leave the ranch for a while, and I . . . Damn it, Reid, you know what I'm trying to say."

"I think so," he replied in a low voice but would not elaborate.

They walked for a few more minutes in silence, both listening to the night. Heather's thoughts reflected again on what she had been thinking during the afternoon at the pond—about her love for Reid and what his true feelings were. Suddenly her resolve to play by his rules faded further, replaced by a need to know the truth, to find the answer to the question she had asked a few minutes ago.

But Heather could not bring herself to repeat the question outright—she was afraid of his answer. When Reid finally turned them in the direction of the house, he spoke.

"I won't be running away. You go ahead and work on your collection. You're an artist as much as I'm a rancher. I'll take care of things for you—you won't have to worry on that account." For Heather there was no comfort in Reid's reassuring words—no comfort, no hope, only a ragged, clawing pain stabbing deeply into her heart.

She whirled on Reid, pulling her hand from his. Her

body ached for him, her need was one of desperation, but at the same time a curtain of ice formed between them.

"No, I won't worry on *that* account, Reid Hunter!" she whispered. Each word was sharp and distinct in the now heavy silence that hung over them. Heather stood, unmoving, as the flood of emotion could no longer be contained. All her doubts about their relationship rose into her mind. All she could do was wait for Reid to speak.

"I don't know what I said to make you angry," he began.

Heather cut off his denial sharply, unwilling to accept his words, but unable to fight him either. "I'm sure you don't. Good night, Reid—I'll see you tomorrow. Maybe then you can try to be honest and open with me." With those parting words Heather turned and fled to her house. Her mind was aflame, but she refused to bend to the threatening onset of tears.

Perhaps he didn't understand, but she couldn't tell him she had not wanted him to say those kind, wonderful words so filled with safety. She wanted him to grab her, to kiss her, to tell her not to go. She wanted to stay with him, here, forever.

But, no, Reid hadn't said he loved her, and she knew he wouldn't. He was a foreman and he wouldn't cross the line, even for love.

Ascending the three steps to the front door, Heather was so upset that she didn't hear the two tall people who had inadvertently walked out from the office when she and Reid had kissed and watched in amazement the fight that they had been unwitting witnesses to.

Chapter Sixteen

Heather could find no solace in sleep, so before any of the ranch hands had risen she was working in her studio. Her hands moved of their own volition, and for the first time in months she let the abstract part of her mind take over. The portion of her brain that guided her talent urged her to express and gave her the ability to create. The form that was taking shape under her fingers was known only to herself, and she was so lost within her endeavors that time did not exist.

Heather was unaware of the fatigue that filled her body—nor did she notice the hunger her empty stomach warned her of. She was only aware of the clay and of what was happening under her fingers.

She also knew that if she stopped working, even for a moment, the memory of last night's debacle would return in full force to destroy the motivation that kept her going.

Heather did not hear her studio door open or even sense Reid's presence behind her as she worked. He stood there for a moment watching her hands move on the clay, fighting the sadness within him. He wanted to touch her, hold her, reassure her, but he couldn't. It would be better if he didn't.

"Heather." She heard him speak but did not acknowledge him. Her hands continued what they were doing while her mind willed him to leave. She could not speak with him—not yet.

"Heather," he said in a louder voice.

"Go away," she whispered.

"I will, but I must talk to you first."

"Talk," she said, fighting back her emotions.

"I won't be less than honest with you. You're an artist, and a damned good one. People everywhere should have the chance to see the work you've created. It would be selfish to keep you to myself. It would also stifle you."

"But what will happen to us?" Heather asked in a low voice, realizing the importance of his answer.

"Nothing. Nothing can happen to us," Reid said, aware that he was hurting her but determined that it must be that way.

Heather held her body still, fighting the trembling that started in her tightly wound nerves. "I thought we had something special. I thought that meant something."

"It means a lot, Heather, but as I told you in the beginning, it can't be."

"How can you say that? How can you stand next to me and say those words? After you've held me, touched me, made love to me . . ."

"I can only tell you how I feel," Reid began, conscious of the harshness of his voice. "The odds are against us. Against you. I tried to tell you before it went too far with us."

"But it did go too far. Reid, you've convinced yourself very well. You're . . . you're a fool! I'm willing to sacrifice for you because I love you. I don't give a damn what anyone has to say about it. I don't care!" Heather told him, her anger gaining over her sensation of deepening loss.

"I'm a fool, I know that. But I'm sacrificing something also, for your own good," Reid said in a whisper. Heather, with a lifetime of relying on her finely tuned senses, disregarded them as she let rage control her.

"Spare me the platitudes. I don't believe in the cowboy's creed. I don't believe in the unspoken rules. I believe in one thing—myself—in the strength I've always had and in what the future holds for me and mine," she said vehemently, no longer hiding the emotions that were clearly written on her face. She was beyond caring whether or not she stepped over the line.

"What is it, Reid? What's holding you back? Don't give me any more stories about your being the foreman and me the boss. It's not that, and we both know it. No more games! Is it because I'm blind? Am I too plain for you?" She suddenly stopped as the shock waves created by her words rippled in her mind.

"I'll leave," Reid said softly. The words echoed in her mind and she knew he meant to leave for good, not just for a few days. Anger rushed through her veins, but this anger was not the red flashing heat that had held her captive seconds ago. This was a cold fury that sped her thoughts with precision and outrage.

"The hell you will! You made me a promise and you signed a contract. You're going to see that promise through. You're not going to walk out on me like you've walked out on your other jobs. I don't care how many ghosts ride on your shoulders, Reid Hunter, you will not walk out on this ranch! I will expect to see you back here within five days to continue what you've begun. And I," Heather said with a sudden softening of her voice, "I will look for a gallery for my first showing."

Heather stopped then, her heart beating fast in her chest, her mind numbed by the fierce emotions she had just vented. She wanted to touch him, to put her fingers on his lips, his eyes, his cheeks, and see what he was thinking. But she couldn't. To touch him would put lies to everything she'd said.

"All right. I won't let the ranch down. Good-bye, Heather. I'll be back in a few days," Reid said as he turned and walked away.

Fighting not to give in to tears, Heather turned back to her workbench and to the clay. But she could not hold her emotions at bay anymore. Too much had happened in the past hours. Heather's hands balled into fists and she began to pummel the clay unmercifully, destroying, in her hurt and ire, what she had created. As this flood tide of emotions was let loose, she cried, tearing, ragged sobs that sounded above the flat echoes of her hands hitting the clay. For an endless time Heather was lost to her emotions, but finally with this powerful outpouring came a new calm.

He was gone, she realized, and not just for the five days. He was lost to her completely. She had tried, but she had failed. She loved and accepted him, but he could not accept himself, she understood suddenly. And she could not fight that. She could battle anything else—anything but that.

She didn't know how long she had stood at the bench, her hands sunk into the misshapen mass of clay, when she realized there were no more tears left to cry. The tears had dried on her face, mixed with the fine dust that permeated the studio. Heather could feel the stiff downward paths the tears had left. She went to the basin and washed. When she had dried her face, she left the studio for the house, not even bothering to cover the destroyed sculpture.

She wanted to be alone, but not alone in the studio. Slowly, she walked to the house, and with each step she forced herself to come to terms with what had happened. She knew the only salvation she had was herself, and the strength that made her believe she would survive. She had done it before, when her mother had died, when her father had died, and she would do it again, now that her love had been taken from her.

"What are you talking about?" Gwen Hunter yelled into the telephone.

Emma stopped what she was doing and glanced at the tall woman. She saw agitation and worry on Gwen's face but forced her eyes away.

"He can't do that! We have a contract. You tell that high-and-mighty son of . . . *Ohhhh!*" Gwen screamed, stopping herself from finishing the words.

This time Emma could not help looking at her.

"You tell him that if he cancels the show he'll never have another showing in the Southwest!"

Emma watched as Gwen stood there, her eyes closed, trying to regain her composure. She watched as she saw the woman's face relax and saw the same lines of determination that she had noticed in Reid's face appear on his sister's. *Uh-oh*, she thought as she hid her smile. She had a feeling of what was coming.

"Laureen, you tell Victor Ainsworth that we do not accept the cancellation of his contract. That's all. Then call John Melville and tell him we want an injunction served on the other gallery the day the show opens, stopping all public and private viewing and sales. Also, find us another artist to fill in for the three weeks. Mr. Ainsworth is going to lose a lot of money along with his friend at Jorgenson's."

Emma shook her head and pulled her eyes from Gwen Hunter as the woman hung up the phone. "Does this mean you'll be leaving us soon?" Emma asked.

"I didn't want to—I haven't had a vacation in three years—but it looks that way," Gwen replied as she moved to Emma's desk. "I own an art gallery in Sante Fe and my premiere artist has just jumped to another gallery."

"There are lots of good artists in Sante Fe and the surrounding areas. Why not use one of them?" Emma asked as an idea formed in her mind.

"Because Victor Ainsworth is becoming a well-known and well-sold artist. This one show could possibly pay my bills for the next year."

"He paints?" Emma asked.

"No, he's a sculptor."

"Abstract?"

"Realist."

"Too bad," Emma said in a falsely sympathetic voice that caught Gwen off guard. Emma disregarded the strange look the dark-haired woman favored her with as she let a smile play on her lips. "I know a sculptor who has no rival anywhere."

"Emma, you've been very nice to me, letting me use the phone to yell and scream. But what I need doesn't grow on the range. Are you familiar with Ainsworth's work?"

"No. I'm only familiar with one artist's work. Gwen, do you speak to your brother frequently?"

"Which one, the prince or the pauper?" she asked bitingly, then, realizing her mistake, she went on quickly. "Excuse me. I'm just in a bitchy mood. I've spoken to Reid twice in the last year. Why?"

"He never told you?" Emma asked, puzzled by Gwen's first remark.

"Told me what?" Gwen asked defensively. Emma read the woman's tone correctly and smiled.

"I'm not trying to pry. Didn't he tell you about Heather?"

"I . . . well, last night I was walking with Tom, and I saw Reid and Heather . . . they were . . ."

"That's not what I . . . Oh, no. Tom saw them?"

"More than saw them! Isn't that what you're talking about?" Gwen asked, her mind whirling from this strangely disjointed conversation.

"No. And please don't let her know she was seen. What I meant was, didn't Reid tell you that Heather is an artist?"

"Not a word," Gwen said. Just then they heard the door at the front of the house close, and both women were silent. After another few moments, when Emma was sure that Heather was safely inside the house, she motioned for Gwen to follow her. Once outside, she turned to Gwen with a smile.

"I think we can solve your problem. When was Ainsworth's show supposed to start?"

"In three weeks," Gwen said with a choking sound of anger.

"That should be enough time."

"Enough time?" Gwen repeated the question as her eyes saw the sculpture-lined walk for the first time. Without another word, Gwen followed Emma into the small adobe building, and when the lights were turned on, her mouth fell open in disbelief.

"As I said, there should be enough time," repeated Emma. Suddenly Emma's eyes went to Heather's workbench and the misshapen mound of clay that sat there. She stared at it for a few minutes before she turned back to Gwen.

"Gwen, I think you'd better tell me exactly what you saw last night."

Heather sat at the kitchen table, moving her fork aimlessly around on the half-eaten plate of food. At her feet was Polaris, who had not left her since she returned to the house. The radio had just informed her that it was seven o'clock, but she didn't care.

A knock on her door interrupted her random thoughts. "It's open," she called.

Heather heard an unfamiliar pattern of footsteps but could tell they were a woman's.

"Good evening," came Gwen Hunter's voice.

"Good evening," Heather replied in a surprised tone. She'd thought Gwen had gone with Reid because of the family problem.

"You didn't know?" Gwen asked.

"No, no one told me you were staying on."

"I hope it's not an inconvenience."

"Of course not," Heather responded, forcing a quick smile to her lips to hide the strain on her face. "Please sit."

"Heather, I won't beat around the bush. Something happened to me today that's knocked me for a loop," Gwen said as she sat on the chair next to Heather.

Heather smiled suddenly.

"Welcome to the club," she said. "Sorry, go on."

"Heather, you're a very talented artist. I had no idea

that someone who was blind could work with the degree of skill you have."

"Thank you, but I don't think being blind has anything to do with skill."

"You'd be surprised," Gwen said with a laugh. "I can't believe this conversation. I can't believe my pigheaded brother either! He never once mentioned you." Heather heard more than just a little anger in the woman's voice.

"Gwen, this is all going over my head. Would you mind explaining?"

"I own an art gallery in Sante Fe. I learned today that my next show has been canceled by the artist."

Heather stood mute as the words rolled through her mind. *"I own a gallery . . ."*

"What are you trying to say?" Heather asked, afraid of what was running through her mind at that instant. The thoughts weren't very pretty.

"I saw some of your work today. You are an extremely talented artist. One of the best I've ever seen," Gwen reiterated, her voice growing stronger as she talked. "I saw the bust of Gregg Farley, and Reid's also. I just couldn't believe my eyes, or my luck."

"Your luck?" Heather asked. A sudden patch of intuition, combined with her words to Reid, told her what was happening, and she began to feel manipulated.

"Heather, I need an artist—not just an artist, but a damn good one. You. I'd like you to come to Sante Fe and let me show your work," Gwen said in a rush of words.

"When I feel I'm ready to give a showing, it will be my decision, and my decision alone!" she stated. "You can tell your brother that I don't need him to find a gallery for me!"

"My brother? What has Reid got to do with this?"

"Don't try to tell me this idea wasn't his," Heather said scathingly.

"Reid's? He didn't even know Ainsworth canceled the showing. In fact, he wouldn't even know who Ainsworth is," she said as she reached across the table and took Heather's hand in hers. Gwen's grip was light, yet firm, as she began to speak again. "Heather, I'd like you to have your first show at my gallery. I don't want to upset you or push you. I just want you to know that I feel you're a very talented artist, and you are ready for a show."

"I . . ." began Heather, unable to think clearly in the jumble that was her mind. Too much had happened in a short time span. Reid, Gwen—it was all coming too fast.

"Please, Heather, I need you. I need an artist of your caliber. And I promise you my brother has no idea that I'm asking you this."

"Victor Ainsworth," Heather said as the familiar name rang in her mind.

"Yes," Gwen said, and told her exactly what had happened.

"But he's one of the best. I couldn't possibly take his place."

"He won't have much of a place when my lawyers finish with him. There won't be many gallery owners who'll want him either. You don't break commitments at the last minute and expect to be welcomed in the art community."

"Gwen, I can't be ready in three weeks," Heather said, already thinking about what she could show.

"If you'll agree to the show, I'll have you ready. Agree!" Gwen ordered in mock command.

"Let me sleep on it," Heather asked.

"Heather."

"Yes?"

"Trust me. You are a great talent."

"Thank you," she said as a wave of warmth for Gwen settled in her mind, a rekindling of the same feeling of friendship she'd had when she first met her.

Chapter Seventeen

Heather slept soundly that night; no dreams disturbed her, no noises bothered her. She woke rested. Listening to the morning sounds of the ranch, Heather felt better. The men walking to the dining room, their voices loud and cheerful, helped to solidify her mood. And Heather knew that as long as she did not think of Reid she would be all right.

When Gwen had left last night, Heather had put her dishes into the sink, told Polaris to run, and had taken a hot bath. As she soaked in the tub, she had tried to organize her thoughts.

She had believed Gwen, believed that Reid had not spoken to her or asked his sister to give Heather a show. She had also wanted to trust Gwen.

In the bath she had been unable to keep her thoughts away from Reid, no matter how hard she tried. Had he arrived safely? Heather had felt her throat constrict as she realized she didn't know where Reid was going. He had never said. Damn him! No more, Heather had decided. She would not play his games anymore. Whatever was bothering Reid, it would be up to him to solve the problem. She had tried. Now she had to think about herself. She had to.

After the bath, Heather had gone to bed. She'd been worried she would be unable to sleep again, but even as she was thinking it, she'd fallen asleep.

Heather stood and stretched and went to the bathroom. When she emerged, her hair was brushed and makeup applied. She dressed in jeans and a cotton top and felt hungry for the first time in two days.

She was standing at the sink, filling the percolator, when she heard Tom Farley's voice carry up from beneath the window.

"Gwen, I really enjoyed myself last night. Would you like to go out for dinner tonight?"

"Thank you, Tom, you're very sweet. I'd love to," Heather heard her say. After almost two days of unhappiness, Heather smiled as she listened to Tom and Gwen. Something had happened between them when they'd met and, whatever it was, Heather liked the way Tom sounded.

By the time the coffee was done, Heather had cooked two eggs and made some toast. She ate quickly, giving in to the demands of her body, but when she was finished, she sat back and drank her coffee slowly. As she was pouring her second cup, she heard Emma enter the office and then come into the kitchen.

"'Mornin', hon. Got an extra cup?"

"You'll condescend to drinking my coffee?" Heather asked in mock horror.

"It'll be hard, but I'll manage."

"I'm sure you will."

"At my age, I've learned how to get by on anything —even your coffee!"

"Heather, did Gwen speak to you?" Emma asked.

"So it was you," Heather said, accusingly.

"Who else would have had the nerve?"

"I thought it had been Reid," Heather admitted.

"Are you going to take this opportunity?"

"I'm thinking about it," she admitted.

"Thinking about it? Don't think! Do!" Heather felt the strength of Emma's words as if they'd been thrown at her. "Don't waste your life here. God gave you a talent rarer than a diamond. Please, hon, please don't waste it."

Heather held her breath as she listened to her friend's words and fought the flood of emotions that washed over her. It had always been her dream, until her father's death, to become a true artist. She had always wanted to spend her days creating the things she loved, so she could have showings where others could see and appreciate the beauty of what she herself could not see with her own eyes. She had suppressed the desire for so long that now she was afraid to think about it.

And Reid? Would there be any chance at all if she left the ranch for a show? No—that had been settled yesterday.

"Heather, you were born to be an artist, not a rancher. Your father knew that. You know it. Reid Hunter is your chance to become!"

"Become what!" she yelled bitterly. Then she sat back, fighting her emotions. "I'm sorry, Emma."

"I . . . it has to be your decision. I just want you to know you've fulfilled your obligations to the ranch and to your father." Emma stopped there, not trusting herself to go further with this discussion. After what she had learned from Gwen yesterday, she could well imagine the turmoil in Heather's mind.

"Thank you, again," Heather said.

"Again?" Emma questioned.

"I can still hear the way you sounded when you told me about yourself. You made me face my own needs."

"Hon, I hope I didn't cause you to do something you're regretting."

She knew, Heather realized suddenly. Somehow Emma knew. "No," she said. "I've nothing to regret." Heather forcefully maintained an even tone in her voice and managed an encouraging smile. "Besides, I don't have time to think about men right now. Not if I've got to get ready for a show in three weeks."

"Really?"

"Really!" Heather stated, understanding she had made the only decision she could. If Gwen thought she was good enough to take the chance of using her to replace a well-known artist, then she had no choice but to agree.

"That's wonderful. . . . My goodness, even your coffee tastes good this morning." Both women laughed at that.

"Emma?" Heather called softly.

"It will work out," Emma said.

"I know. What's going on between Tom and Gwen?"

"How'd you find out already?"

"I heard them talking this morning."

"You're turning into a peeping Tom," Emma admonished.

"They were standing under my window."

"It's no secret. I think Tom Farley fell head over heels in love with her the minute he saw her. And she's nice, too," Emma added.

"But she's not a rancher. I think maybe Tom's going to get hurt again."

"Neither was Tom until five years ago—don't forget that," Emma reminded her. "Besides, that's Tom's business, and you have enough problems to keep you busy. Let them work out theirs by themselves."

"Yes, ma'am," Heather replied.

"Now, I'll get Gwen so you can give her the news."

The sun was setting; the change in the air told Heather that fact. The July heat had grown strong, but the evenings were a blessed relief. It had been hot in the studio as she, Gwen, and one of the men had finished the last of the packing. For four days Heather and Gwen had worked continually, sorting, picking, choosing, only to reject all their choices and begin again, until at last they made their final decisions. They chose fifteen pieces in all: four busts, four animal figures, and seven large abstract pieces. The abstracts were the ones that Gwen felt would bring the highest praise from the critics.

"Heather," Gwen said, taking a deep breath and wiping the perspiration from her forehead, "I've made all the arrangements. The freight company will be here tomorrow, and in three days everything will arrive in Sante Fe. No," Gwen said cutting off Heather's next remark. "Everything will be fine. The shipping company is the only one I use. They specialize in art works. You don't have to worry about that."

"I can't help it. I guess I'm nervous," she admitted.

"Don't be. The pieces will be safe and you'll be a big hit. The first press releases were sent to the papers yesterday."

"Gwen, what press releases?" After four days of working closely with Gwen, Heather had found out how little she knew about the other end of the art business.

"I spoke with my assistant right after you agreed to the show. I gave her your background and she wrote up several releases, which were sent to the papers. If the newspapers are interested, they print them, and most interview you when you get to Sante Fe."

Heather listened and digested everything Gwen told her. "Do you think they'll be interested?"

"Heather, they'll have no choice. If only to see the work that's replacing Ainsworth's."

"And to laugh at a blind artist's perceptions?"

"No."

"How can you be so sure?" Heather asked.

"Because no one will be told you're blind until after opening night."

Heather felt tears of love build in her eyes at Gwen's words. This was something she had not expected. She'd expected a big deal to be made out of the fact that she was blind.

"Th . . . thank you," she mumbled. Then she felt the tall woman's arms around her and put her own around Gwen.

"You're welcome. Now don't make me cry. You're a wonderful artist, blind or not. Don't forget that."

"I'll try not to."

"Good. Come to dinner with Tom and Gregg and myself tonight?" Gwen asked.

Heather felt a momentary loss but shrugged it away. "I'd love to," she said with a smile.

"Okay. Let's double-check these last three crates and then we can clean up."

Less than an hour later Heather stood under her shower. Washing the grime and dust from her skin, she smiled at the thought of the friendship that was growing so strong between her and Gwen. Gwen was so open, so warm, and so giving that Heather had found it difficult not to question her background and learn more about Reid. But she had fought the impulses, deciding that what she did not know would make it easier for her to accept the loss of the man she loved.

By the time she had finished her shower and dressed, everyone was ready. Heather sat in the back seat with Gregg, while Tom and Gwen sat up front. Not only was Heather hungry, but she was looking forward to having company while she ate dinner.

Suddenly another thought struck her. How was Gregg taking this new situation with his father and Gwen? Tomorrow, Heather decided, she would have a talk with Gregg. She wasn't trying to be nosy—she just loved the boy and wanted him to be happy.

Sitting back and letting the cool evening air rush across her face, Heather smiled. In two days she would be gone. She and Gwen would drive to Reno and fly to Albuquerque and then drive to Santa Fe. Even with the hurt of losing Reid in her mind, a new excitement was growing strongly within her. She had been waiting for a long time for this opportunity, and now she found she wanted it very badly.

She would be staying with Gwen at her home, and in a few days the present exhibit at the Hunter Gallery would close. During the next week she and Gwen would set up for her show.

Her first show! Her unveiling, she thought.

Chapter Eighteen

$\mathcal{A}$re you sure I have everything?" Heather asked, doubt filling her voice and making it quaver slightly.

"Everything, right down to your panty hose," Emma replied. "You're all set. Even Polaris has his ticket and his bowls. Relax. Go for a walk. It will help you calm down. You're as nervous as Tom is upset."

"How bad is he?"

"He's hurting, but he'll survive. I heard him make plane reservations for the show. He's going to be there opening night. And I don't think it's only because of you."

"No," agreed Heather, "I don't think so either. He sure did fall hard."

"So did Gwen. She's as down and out as he is."

"I'm glad."

"You would be. I think there're some very good possibilities for those two. It'll take time. And," Emma added, "Gregg likes her a lot."

"I know. I had a talk with Gregg yesterday. He does like her, and that makes me feel good."

"Hon," Emma began. Heather heard the change in her voice and knew what was coming. "How are you?"

"Honestly?"

"No other way," Emma said.

"I'm surviving. I have to. I haven't spoken to Reid since he got back today. I don't know if I want to," Heather admitted. "It hurts a lot."

"I know. Maybe your leaving will help."

"Help? Being a thousand miles away can't possibly help."

"You can never tell. Maybe he'll realize what he's losing," Emma told her.

"Or maybe he'll breathe easier when I'm gone."

"Maybe," Emma responded. "Now, everything's done. You go take a walk."

"Yes, ma'am!" Heather said as she saluted and left the room. She would miss Emma very much, but she also knew she was being given a wonderful opportunity, one that she'd wanted almost her entire life.

The night air was warm and pleasant as Heather strolled along. Polaris was at her side, pressing against her every so often, more to remind her that he was there than to guide her around the familiar land.

She passed the corral, pausing to listen to the stallion within. She stepped to the rail and cooed to him. A moment later, the large bay came over to her outstretched hand and nuzzled it affectionately.

"Hi, fella. Like your new home?" she asked.

"He should—he's the new king," said Reid. Heather jumped at the sound of his voice, startled that she had not heard him approach.

"Sorry—didn't mean to scare you."

"It's okay," Heather replied, fighting to regain her equilibrium. Along with the surprise had come another rush of emotion, making her mind spin numbly.

"I understand Gwen discovered your talents and is stealing you away from the ranch."

"Not quite stealing. Did you get your problem taken care of?" she asked, trying to regain her poise.

"Everything's settled," he replied. Heather noticed the curt way he spoke and decided again not to pry. She heard Reid take a deep breath and felt the heat radiating from his body. She willed herself to relax, but failed.

"Heather, I'm sorry for the way things turned out. I really am. But it just couldn't happen."

"Why, Reid? At least be honest with me now. I'll be gone in the morning and you won't see me for at least six weeks, maybe longer. Please talk to me. Tell me why."

Reid looked at her, gazed at the face he had missed so much while he was in Albuquerque, and forced his mouth to work.

"It's simple. It's so simple it's hard. Heather, I have nothing. I live a life that takes me from place to place and I do the work I love. But I have nothing to bring into our relationship. You own this ranch. I have nothing to bring to balance the difference. I can't live off of you. I just can't accept that."

Heather listened intensely. She heard what he thought of as their predicament. She also heard the pain. Lifting her arm slowly, Heather reached out and caressed his cheek. "You're wrong, Reid. Very wrong. You have the one thing that's more important."

"What?" Reid asked as his hand covered hers.

"That's what you have to learn. Reid, I love you, but

that doesn't seem to be enough for you. Take care of the ranch," she said as she pulled back her hand and walked away.

Reid watched her go, his mind puzzled. Then, from the corner of his eye, he saw Tom and his sister. He thrust away the haunting thoughts that had invaded his mind and went over to them.

"Evening, Reid," Tom said with a smile.

"Evening, Tom. Mind if I steal my sister for a few minutes?"

"So long as you return her," Tom bandied as he walked away from them, moving toward the spot where Reid and Heather had been only moments before.

"Gwen, watch out for her," Reid said.

"I plan to. Reid, what's wrong with you?"

"What are you talking about?" he asked evasively.

"No games. I think you've about run out of them. I saw what happened the night before you left. I saw and heard it all. So did Tom."

"I suppose you told everyone?" he asked, stunned by his sister's words.

"You don't give me much credit, do you? No, Reid, your secret's safe. Tom knows but he won't say anything. He even likes you."

"Gwen . . ."

"When's it going to end? Reid, when are you going to stop hurting the people who love you?"

"I don't want to hurt anyone, Gwen. I don't," Reid told her. He gazed into his sister's eyes and saw himself reflected there. "Take care of her, please," he finished. Turning, Reid walked away, his shoulders straight, his head held high and unmoving.

"My Lord, it's hot here," Heather said as she opened the car door.

"Just wait until tonight. It'll make your ranch feel like the midday desert. Nights in Santa Fe are chilly," Gwen told her. "Let me take you inside and then I'll get the bags."

"Don't be silly. I'm blind, but I'm not crippled. I can carry my own bags. Do you think the truck got here yet?" Heather asked in a quick rush of words. Ever since the truck had picked up the sculptures she'd been worried. Gwen told her it was natural—all artists felt the same way. Heather couldn't know from experience but empathized with her peers if they went through what she was going through now.

"Stop it!" Gwen admonished as she handed Heather two suitcases. "I suppose Polaris can carry his own bag, too," she said in jest.

"Just hold it for him and say, 'Take,'" Heather told her with a smile. Gwen did just that and laughed delightedly when Polaris took the bag that held his two bowls.

"Okay, follow me," she said.

"Gwen . . ."

"Sorry. Walk straight. I'll tell you when to stop." Heather stopped when Gwen told her to. She put her bags down and waited until the door was open. Then, with Gwen taking one arm, Heather lifted a suitcase and let Gwen guide her inside. The air was cool and fresh without any trace of mustiness.

"Laureen, my assistant, came by this morning and aired the place out. Now wait here until I get the rest of the things."

Heather waited, content to smell the new scents and to think for a moment. The flight from Reno to Albuquerque had been pleasant. They had flown coach and had taken three seats. Heather was on the aisle, Gwen next to her, and Polaris in the window seat. She refused to allow Polaris to be caged and put in the cargo compartment. Because she was blind, the airline did not protest, even as large as the shepherd was.

In Albuquerque Gwen had retrieved her car and they had driven straight to Sante Fe and Gwen's house. For the entire hour's ride, Gwen had kept up a running commentary about the countryside and the people populating it.

Now that she had a moment alone, Heather realized that Gwen had kept up the conversation since the very minute they'd left Tom at the gate and boarded the plane. First it was art and then a guided tour of the New Mexican countryside. Was Gwen trying to make Heather feel better or herself, when she'd left Tom? she wondered.

"All set," Gwen said as the front door closed. "Your bedroom is straight down this hall, on the left." As Gwen spoke, Heather's arm was gripped by Gwen's hand and again she was being guided along. Inside the guest bedroom, Gwen explained the room's layout, and after Heather was unpacked, Gwen took her on a slow tour of the house so that she could learn her new quarters.

Polaris was at her side at all times and he, too, learned the house. "Now, would you like something to drink or a shower?"

"Both!" Heather declared.

"In that case, first a drink to celebrate your arrival and then a shower to get the New Mexican grit off your skin."

As they drank a glass of cold wine, the telephone rang. Gwen answered it, and after she hung up, she turned to Heather. "That was Laureen. The truck arrived safely. It's parked at the gallery, and first thing tomorrow morning you and I will supervise the unloading."

Heather breathed a sigh of relief and smiled at her friend. "Thank you."

"It's all part of my job. Now, let's take our showers and go to dinner. You do like Mexican food?"

"I like food period," Heather said with a laugh.

An hour and a half later, Heather and Gwen arrived at the restaurant. With Gwen's help in choosing her outfit, Heather wore a cinnamon-colored cotton dress and tan shoes. She had done her hair up, tied in a small knot in the back, and wore a single gold chain around her neck. She had meticulously applied her makeup, using her favorite blue shadow and just the lightest hint of blush on her cheeks. The small tan clutch rested comfortably in the crook of her arm.

As they entered the restaurant a momentary hush fell on Heather's ears. She did not know the reason and felt self-conscious but did not show it as they were led to a table and seated. Gwen graciously guided her to the waiting chair before she sat.

"Drinks?" asked the maître d'.

"Heather?"

"White wine," Heather responded.

"The same," said Gwen. Just as Gwen started to say something to Heather, she stopped. "Watch it, here comes trouble." Heather felt someone step next to the table.

"Gwen, darling, I was shattered to hear about Ainsworth. Whatever are you going to do?"

Heather heard the woman's falsely sad tones and mentally cringed for her friend.

"Ainsworth. . . . My goodness, Alicia, it was a relief to have him go. I was waiting for a break so that I could bring a really talented artist in."

"Oh? Who is it?"

"I'll send you an invite, dear—have no fear." Heather almost lost the laugh she was holding back at Gwen's perfect imitation of the woman's voice.

When the woman left, the noise level inside the restaurant picked up again. The drinks were served and menus placed on the table.

"I thought everyone stopped talking because they were watching me," Heather admitted.

"You're not that beautiful," Gwen said.

"No, because I'm—"

"No," Gwen said, cutting her off. "You're not the first blind person or the most beautiful to come here. They were surprised to see me in public. Everyone knows that Ainsworth was under exclusive contract to me in Santa Fe. Jumping to another gallery is supposed to shame the loser."

"But not you," Heather stated.

"I was raised differently. When you have two older brothers, you learn how not to be embarrassed by anything. Also, I didn't introduce you to Miss Bitch for a reason. I'll explain it later. Now, what do you like to eat?"

"Food. You order," Heather told her as she sat back and listened to the voices floating around her. By the time dinner was finished, Heather had learned a great deal more about the tightly knit art community she was now in the midst of.

Some things she liked, other things she would have to get used to. The constant flow of people from table to table, the myriad conversations that flew overhead, and the atmosphere of camaraderie mixed with barely contained jealousy, hate, and small portions of love—all combined to tire Heather and make her even more excited at being with them.

"What would you like to do now?" Gwen asked.

"Now?" Heather replied as she touched her watch. It was almost ten. The strain of the long day was weighing down her mind. "Go to sleep?" she asked in a low voice.

"That's not too bad an idea," Gwen replied as she stood.

"The check?" Heather asked as she reached for her purse.

"I've already signed it."

"But . . ."

"No arguments. We'll settle everything when the time comes. Don't forget, I'm going to make a lot of money from your show."

"Maybe."

"Definitely. Now, shall we get some of that sleep you just mentioned? We've got a big day ahead of us tomorrow."

"Definitely," Heather mimicked with a smile.

Chapter Nineteen

*H*eather threw herself completely into the new world she had entered. By day she worked on preparing her show and by night she became Gwen's shadow.

Again, on the second night out, Gwen did not introduce her to any of the people who came to the table. Gwen had told her, at home that first night, that it was a game to make the other gallery people work hard at finding out what she had up her sleeve. If she had introduced Heather, then their curiosity would not grow. She wanted Heather to remain a mystery until opening night.

Heather had joined in the game, and whenever anyone came to their table, she studiously ignored them, pretending to look elsewhere.

But at night, when she was in her bed waiting for sleep to overtake her, her thoughts drifted to Nevada, to the ranch, and to Reid. No matter how hard she tried to avoid it, she couldn't.

The first two weeks passed quickly, and Heather realized that within a few days the opening would take place. It was still like a dream in her mind—a scary, wonderful dream come true. If only, she thought, the rest of her dream could come to life with it, she would be content.

Heather sat on the edge of the bed, tired from another long day yet feeling no need to sleep. Again tonight she and Gwen had gone out to dinner. Once more Heather had felt the whirlpool of night life surround her with its gaiety and charged atmosphere. But tonight she had realized she was tiring of it quickly.

It was not the life she was used to, and she wondered how the artists who lived this hectic way were able to sustain the quality of their work. After two weeks of riding this merry-go-round, Heather felt drained.

Polaris laid his head on Heather's lap, bringing a smile to her face. "Are you getting tired also?" she asked him as she scratched behind his ear. She heard him exhale deeply, as if in agreement, and dropped her cheek to rest on his soft furry head. When she lifted her head, she heard the doorbell ring, and a moment later heard the echo of Gwen's front door closing.

Standing, Heather went to her door to close it so that both she and Gwen could have their privacy. With her hand on the doorknob she froze as a chill of recognition ran the length of her spine. Polaris heard the voice, too, and tried to go to its source.

It couldn't be, she thought as her fingers dug into Polaris's fur, holding him back. With her breath turning shallow, she listened to the voices arguing only a few yards away.

"You had no right!" came the deep authoritative voice she thought belonged to Reid Hunter. She listened, stunned, as he continued. "You had no right to go to him!"

"I had every right. He's my brother. He's your brother, too. You needed his help, but you wouldn't ask. You wouldn't ask me or him, so I did it for you," Gwen replied, her voice as loud as his.

"So you went to him in order for that high-and-mighty bastard who walked out on us ten years ago to come back and throw it in my face?"

"Stop it! You sound like a child."

"I don't care how I sound. Do you know how it feels to work day in and day out, to do everything you can, and find that what you've worked so hard to build is falling down around your feet?"

"If I didn't, I wouldn't have gone to him," Gwen defended.

"I bet he's laughing right now. Do you know what he did? Of course you do. You signed that damn paper, didn't you?"

"Patrick, will you please calm down." Heather heard the name and her mind reeled with the impact. Patrick, Gwen had called him. Not Reid, but Patrick. He sounded so much like Reid she hadn't been able to tell the difference. Except now that she thought about it, she'd never heard Reid raise his voice—ever.

"Why? After ten years Reid comes back, walks into the house, hands me a piece of paper, and says he's sorry I'm having troubles. Then turns around and tries to leave."

"And of course you stopped him. You told him to take his paper and to . . ."

"That's right. That's just what I told him. I don't need his arrogance. I don't need help from someone who walked out on his family."

"He didn't walk out. Pat, you pushed him out when he wanted understanding. We both did. He didn't want to leave, not permanently. You gave him no choice. But you knew that, and that's why you didn't give him back the paper."

"I gave him plenty of choices. He picked the wrong one. And now he has the audacity to come to me and try to help me? Do you know what he did?" Patrick repeated.

"Yes," Gwen replied. "He gave you our permission to mortgage the ranch. He gave you a way to raise enough money and to prevent you from selling any more of Broadlands land. But you can't handle that, can you?" yelled Gwen, taking the offensive now. "No," she continued, her voice growing stronger as she pressed on, "when it was Reid who was available to take the blame for things, you let him. But you can't face your own mistakes. You made one bad decision— just one—and when we offer you help, you can't handle it."

"Help? Do you call what he did help? He walked into the house, looked at me, and said he was sorry to hear I was having trouble. Then he handed me the paper and told me it would be a good idea if I went to the bank. He said it would be *best* not to sell off any more land. Then he turned around and walked out," Patrick finished.

"No he didn't," Gwen stated. "I know you both. You're both stubborn. Reid waited for you to say something, anything. But you didn't, did you?"

"I had nothing to say."

"You could have said thank you," Gwen told him in a low, tear-filled voice.

Heather's mind staggered under the wealth of information that was being forced into it. She needed time to accept and understand it. What was happening? What?

Heather could not move. She was rooted to the spot. Suddenly the voices stopped and she heard the front door slam, followed by Gwen's footsteps on the tile floor of the hallway. She knew Gwen was coming toward her, but still she could not move.

"Oh! Heather!" Gwen said, stopping within inches of her. "I . . . I'm sorry you had to hear that."

Heather could find no words to answer Gwen. She was still too stunned by what had happened—too shocked and too hurt. She had been deceived by Reid, and by Gwen also. The tension and stiffness in her body made her rigid. Slowly, she willed order into the confusion that was her mind, and gradually, over an eternity, she began to breathe again.

"Heather . . ." Gwen began.

"No," she said immediately, the word cold and cutting as it echoed in the hallway. "Right now all I want is the truth. No more lies, no more stories. I thought you were my friend. I trusted you. I've taken your advice and I've listened to you. Now I want some answers, and I want the *truth!*" she demanded as rage filled her mind.

"Heather, I promised Reid."

"I don't give a damn about what you promised Reid!" Releasing her hold on Polaris, Heather crossed her arms on her chest. She fought away the emotions of betrayal and kept her anger in check, waiting.

"All right, Heather, but can we at least sit down? It's not a short story," she sighed.

After they were seated in the living room, Gwen began to speak. She spoke for an hour, and when she was done her cheeks were soaked with tears.

"And that's why things turned out this way," she finished.

Heather was silent, trying to put it all into perspective. But her anger would not allow it. She was incensed by Reid Hunter's pride and his deceit. Slowly, Heather rose. She took a deep breath before she spoke.

"You do know about Reid and me?" Heather asked. She received silence. "Gwen?" Gwen's light laughter, bordering on the hysterical, filled the room. "Gwen?"

"I'm sorry. Yes, I know," she said, and told Heather about what she and Tom had seen.

"Why did Reid tell me we could never have a life together because he was just a cowboy and I owned a ranch? Why did he lie if he loves me?"

"He didn't lie. He doesn't own any part of the ranch. I told you that he signed over his rights to the ranch when he left ten years ago. Well, he did, but he did not give up his inherited ownership of the ranch—only the monies derived from it."

"I understand that," Heather said, still controlling the hurt that kept burrowing deeper into her heart. "But that still means he lied to me."

"Yes and no. When he went to Albuquerque and saw Patrick, he gave Patrick something from both of us. He gave Patrick a legal agreement, deeding to him sole title to Broadlands. In order to get Patrick out of the trouble he was in, Reid and I agreed to relinquish all claims to Broadlands. In effect, we signed over title so he could mortgage the property. Our father put a stipulation in his will that stated that as long as more than one sibling retained ownership, the land could not be mortgaged. Reid felt there was only one way Pat could get out from under, and we both agreed.

"When Reid returned to your ranch, he had nothing left of his past life. He had just given up the only thing that might possibly have salved his pride enough to bring himself to marry you," Gwen finished.

"What makes you or him think I would even consider marriage," Heather spat suddenly. "Marriage means trust! You can't love and marry someone who lies to you."

"He didn't think he had any choice," pleaded Gwen, still vainly trying to defend her brother.

Suddenly Heather needed to be outside to breathe the sweet, fresh air of the night. With Polaris at her side Heather strode from the living room. She walked to the rear of the adobe house and out the back door. Stepping into the cool New Mexican night, Heather walked to the bench that was in the center of Gwen's garden. She wanted to be alone, to think, to understand what had happened to her life and to try and bury her love so she could rid herself of the awful pain that was tearing her apart.

Chapter Twenty

Reid sat on the split-wood fence that surrounded the original Strand homestead. His eyes were fixed on a rabbit twenty feet away. The rabbit sat up; its eyes searched the area around it warily. It bolted suddenly as Reid lit a cigarillo. His hazel eyes followed the animal until it disappeared behind the pointed tufts of a small clump of sagebrush.

Reid's eyes stayed fixed on the spot where the rabbit had disappeared, but they didn't see the sagebrush; they saw nothing at all. His mind had not registered what his eyes had seen. Reid's thoughts were a thousand miles from Nevada.

It had been two weeks since he'd last seen Heather, he thought as he took another deep inhalation of smoke. Then, as he exhaled, he hopped down from the fence and forced away the thought that came chasing on the heels of his first one. He walked around, trying to think about the camp that would be here next summer, trying to picture the children who would be here, learning, playing, and enjoying life.

But it didn't work. He wanted to enjoy life too. He wanted to ride this land, not alone as he had today but with the woman he had ridden with months ago to this very spot.

Reid could still picture Heather as she rode the gelding, her head bent close to the horse's neck as she urged him along the plateau on that clear and cloudless day. The smile that had radiated over her face had filled him with unspoken joy.

Then Reid remembered the last times he and Heather had talked—fought, actually. He had tried to make her understand what was driving him, but she would not listen. When in desperation he told her he'd leave, she wouldn't let him do that either. "You're not walking out on this ranch, Reid Hunter!" she'd said. Her face had been set in grim lines of determination and Reid had known he would be unable to go.

Those last words she'd said to him bothered him more than anything else. "You have the one thing that is more important," she'd told him. Reid had spent the last lonely weeks trying to figure out what she'd meant.

Stopping himself from further thought, Reid crushed the cigarillo beneath his boot and turned around. Slowly, like a drill bit biting into rock, he started to comprehend what Heather had said. He began to walk purposefully toward his horse.

Reid untied the horse from the fence, but before he mounted it he looked again at the old house that had been built by one of Heather's pioneering ancestors. In the five months he'd been here, Heather Strand had turned his well-ordered life around and made him question the basic commitments that had been relentlessly driving him.

Yes, suddenly Reid knew what it was he had been searching for all these years. He knew what he wanted and where it was. He had known it on that first night he and Heather had spent together, the night they had shared themselves with each other and become one. But until now he had not permitted himself to think about it, or believe it would be possible.

Slipping his foot into the stirrup, Reid mounted his horse. With a flick of his wrist, he turned the animal and started back to the ranch and his office.

Reid Hunter had a phone call to make.

Heather sat on the cotton-weave couch in Gwen's living room, sipping iced tea and fighting to keep her mind focused on the path she had set. Last night in the garden she had sat for many hours, thinking, crying, and reassessing her needs. What she had learned last night had nearly devastated her.

The words Patrick Hunter had spoken and the truth Gwen had revealed took from her the one hope she had been nurturing since she'd stepped onto the plane in Nevada—her hope that Reid would not give up on their love. But last night she had realized he would give it up. Their love had been founded on lies, half-truths, and deception.

Heather knew she must pick herself up as she had always done and, by herself, keep her life going. At one point last night Gwen had come out to the garden and sat next to her. Reid's sister had been silent for a long time, but finally she had spoken.

"I am sorry, Heather—more so than you can imagine. I'm sorry you had to learn about Reid in this way. But, he is my brother and I love him. In the short time we've known one another I've grown to love you also. I don't know whether you believe me or not, but hiding the truth from you was tearing me apart. I don't like being dishonest, but I kept hoping it would be Reid who would tell you the truth."

Heather had not replied right away. She had listened to what Gwen had to say and had thought about it. She remembered the instant sensation of friendship she'd experienced and the trust her instincts had told her to place in the woman. Had that, too, been because of her feelings for Reid? No, it had been because she liked Gwen Hunter as her own person.

While she had sat there thinking, she'd heard Gwen take a deep breath, stand, and begin to walk away.

"Wait," she had called. "Gwen, you're not to blame. I know you were caught in the middle and I know you're my friend."

A moment later, she had felt Gwen's arms go around her, pulling her into a close embrace. "I wish I could help you," Gwen had said in a choked voice. "I wish I could."

Strangely, Heather had begun to feel worse for Gwen than for herself. Her arms had gone around her friend and she had comforted the tall woman. Nothing else had been said—there had been no need. A few minutes later, Gwen had drawn away and left Heather to her solitude.

She'd spent a good portion of the night sitting on the bench, unresponsive to the cold night air, while Polaris had lain uncomplaining at her feet. Finally her mind had begun to settle and she had started to block out some of the hurt. It would take time, she had realized—time, work, and effort—to rid herself of the love she felt for Reid Hunter.

She had also taken the time to reinforce her resolve to build her career. From this moment forward, Heather had told herself, she would not make the same mistake. She had given herself twice, and twice she had been rejected. She would accept no more rejection. From this point on Heather was determined to dedicate herself to her art and to give all her love to it.

"You must be exhausted," Gwen said as she sat next to Heather, bringing her mind back from last night.

"I'm not allowed to be. We have another night of dining and partying awaiting us," Heather remarked, trying to bring some humor into her voice.

"We did, but I thought you might not want to because . . ."

"Because?" Heather prompted at Gwen's hesitation.

"Well, after last night I didn't think you'd be in a very sociable mood."

"Thank you—you're right. But I think I do want to go out," she said, preferring a crowd to a lonely room.

"You're not too tired?"

"An elephant would be tired having to keep up with you!" Heather declared.

"But it was for the best, wasn't it?"

"I'm still mad at you for sneaking in that interview."

"Be mad, but smile, because that interview is going to make you a lot of money. Now, if you'll excuse me, I have some calls to make."

"Tom?" Heather asked.

"First Laureen—I have to check on the final details of the party. We only have until tomorrow at seven to have everything ready. Then Tom."

"Will many people come?" Heather asked. She still couldn't believe that her first showing would draw the crowd Gwen had said it would.

"After all the publicity we received because of Ainsworth's cancellation and the mysterious circumstances surrounding my new 'discovery,' I'd say just about everyone who is anyone will be there."

"Oh . . ." Heather said as the sudden thought of many strangers crowding around her turned her heart cold.

"Don't worry—you're going to be a success!"

"At least in that department," Heather whispered to Gwen's retreating footfalls.

"I thought you didn't believe in self-pity," Gwen said suddenly, her voice whiplike in Heather's ears.

"It wasn't self-pity," Heather stated. "Just fact."

"Oh, please," Gwen shot back just before she closed the door to her den.

"It wasn't self-pity," Heather said to the empty room as the sudden memory of her fingers on Reid's face floated into her mind. She could "see" the cutting edges of his strong chin and the slight bump on his nose. *No!* she ordered herself. *Think of something else—anything else.*

Heather leaned her head back on the couch's cushions, closed her eyes, and in her effort to avoid thinking of Reid she thought about the fast-paced morning and afternoon she had just had.

She thought about the breakfast she had not tasted, her mind still filled with the painful memory of last night, which the three hours of sleep she'd finally gotten had been unable to wash away. She'd gone with Gwen to the boutique to try on the dress, to see if any additional alterations were needed.

A week ago, Gwen had brought up the subject of what Heather would wear for her opening. Heather hadn't realized she needed to be dressed up, but Gwen insisted she dress in style. Gwen had wanted Heather to wear an evening gown. Heather had argued she was not the gown type and would feel uncomfortable. At the boutique Gwen had taken her to, Heather chose a dress that was stylish, elegant, yet not quite as formal as Gwen's first choice.

"It's your night, Heather," Gwen had told her on the first visit to the store. "You're the one who'll be on center stage. You should dress the part."

"I can't dress a part that's not me," she had replied. "I'm going to be nervous enough. At least let me feel comfortable with what I have on."

Gwen had acquiesced reluctantly, and at this morning's final fitting she had grudgingly admitted Heather had been right. The dress looked perfect on her, and Gwen had told her that she did indeed look comfortable and well dressed. The only problem Heather had during the final fitting was wondering if the dress was *too* much for her.

Then they had gone to lunch at a quaint Mexican restaurant on the outskirts of Santa Fe. During the drive Gwen described the varied adobe houses they passed, as well as the people who occupied them. Names of famous artists and writers had flown from Gwen's lips and Heather had felt a thrill race through her at their mention. She had wondered if at some point another person would feel the same way when *her* name was mentioned.

After a delicious lunch that Heather had barely touched—a fact Gwen had tactfully not mentioned—they had driven back to town, where without warning Gwen had taken her to her first interview.

"But you said not until the show opened," Heather had protested while she tried to untwist the knot that had formed in her stomach.

"I know. But this one is different," Gwen had replied. "The Santa Fe *Voice* is a weekly magazine, and if we want to get into the next issue, we have to do the interview today. It won't be published until your show is a week old. And besides, in return for giving them this interview and an early private viewing they have promised not to speak to any of the other media people about you."

"It's not fair," Heather had protested again.

"It's how you play the game."

"No, I mean to me."

"Would you rather I had told you about it last week and let you worry?" Gwen had asked in a gentle tone.

"I guess not. But why are they interviewing me before they see my work?" Heather had asked. Gwen's silence had answered her. "When?"

Gwen had laughed softly before she answered. "They were at the gallery this morning. Laureen gave them a preview while you were being fitted. Here we are," she said as she pulled to the curb. "Relax. Answer the questions freely and be yourself."

Heather had taken Gwen's advice and, after the first few minutes, she relaxed, secure in the knowledge that the interviewer was both experienced in his craft and very good at it. The interview had lasted over an hour, and when it was finished, Heather had the distinct impression that the journalist was satisfied also.

The magazine's art critic had come in at the end of the interview session and talked with Heather for a few minutes. He told her he was impressed with her work but would not elaborate further. He asked about her favorite artists, and they discussed each other's likes and dislikes.

In the car Gwen had laughed. "They loved your work. I spoke to Laureen. He was raving about it when he left. Laureen reminded him of the magazine's promise. Neither the critic nor the writer will tell anyone until the show opens. Now," Gwen had said as her voice turned serious, "I think it's time to call it a day."

"Heather?" Gwen called softly, "are you awake?" Gwen's voice pulled Heather from the place she'd escaped to and brought her back to the living room.

"I'm afraid I am."

"I have to go out. Laureen is having a problem with the caterer. I won't be long, and when I get back, I'll fix us some dinner."

"Don't rush. How was Tom?" Heather asked.

"He wasn't in. I talked to Gregg—he said to say 'hi,' and he can't wait until tomorrow." Heather smiled at Gwen, a warm feeling settling in her mind as she listened to Gregg's message. Gwen left and silence descended again in the house. Heather did not feel like moving. A grip of lethargy held her within its grasp and she could not summon the energy to break it. She tried not to think of Reid, but she failed at that also.

Heather knew she must use logic to fight the ache in her heart. She must use rationalities to chase away the memories of his touch, his lips, and his soft and gentle words.

Haunting memories of their many nights of love rushed through her mind with a paralyzing force that held her captive, and Heather's emotions rose to the breaking point. Clenching her fists, Heather fought herself until the shrill ringing of the telephone broke her concentration.

She didn't want to answer the phone—not in her state of mind—but she had to. She was a guest in Gwen's house and the call might be important. Slowly, she picked up the telephone from the table next to the couch.

"Hello?" Heather asked.

"Heather?" Heather felt her body become as rigid as rock at the sound of Reid Hunter's voice.

"Yes," she whispered.

"How are you?" he asked in his deep, soft voice.

How am I? she repeated in her mind. "How should I be?" she snapped back.

"Is something wrong?" Reid asked, his tone conveying his bewilderment at her words.

"Yes, damn it, something's wrong—you're wrong!" she yelled, unable to hold in her rush of anger, unable to control her emotions after hearing the voice she had dreamed of for weeks. All her work, all the effort she had spent in submerging her feelings since last night, had become wasted. With Reid on the telephone she could no longer hold herself back.

"You lied to me. From the beginning you deceived and tricked me. Did you have fun? Is that what you really do with your life? Go from ranch to ranch and make women fall in love with you, and when they do, you move on to greener pastures? Is that what happened at the Triple-K?" she asked, not bothering to think out her words. Heather was past caring, past worrying about the ramifications of what she said.

"No, Heather, you're wro—"

"Don't say another word to me. I can't listen to any more of your lies. I loved you! Do you understand? I gave you all of my love. I would have given you anything you asked for, anything. I loved you with all my heart," she said, her voice dropping to a hoarse whisper, "but all you gave me were lies."

"Listen to me," Reid yelled, his voice exploding from the receiver.

"I've listened to all the excuses and explanations I'm going to. Reid Hunter, you are a selfish, unreliable, and . . . and . . . and as rotten a bastard as I've ever known! I want you out of my life! I don't want to hear about your grief-stricken conscience or your pious deeds. I know all about the way you walked out on your brother and on your birthright. I know all about your stupid damned pride, and I don't want to know anything more!" she said as she slammed down the phone.

"Oh . . . no," she cried as her hands came up and cupped her face. "Oh, Reid, why?" she asked.

Years passed that night and Heather was still in the same position. She had replayed the phone call a hundred times, and no matter how she repeated her harsh words in her mind, she knew she could have done nothing else. She still loved him, she realized—her angry and irrational screaming had only proved the truth of that—but the yelling she'd done represented a release, a catharsis her mind had needed.

She had told him the source of her pain, what he had done to her. She had told him and had been freed. No, she thought, not freed, but under a new control. She would be able to go on with her life, alone, but with the knowledge that she had been truthful.

Slowly, without realizing it, Heather slid down on the couch and fell into a dreamless sleep. She did not move when Gwen came home, nor did she feel the blanket that she was covered with. She didn't even hear how hard Gwen had to pull Polaris to get him to leave Heather to go out for his walk.

She slept soundly, peacefully, and deeply.

Chapter Twenty-one

The hum from Gwen's office air conditioner seemed to match the hum inside Heather's head and body. But even those two distinct vibrations could not mask the sounds of the final preparations for tonight's opening party.

Heather smiled. Gwen had once again kept her moving through the day in an effort, Heather knew, to keep her mind off Reid and also to help speed the day and ease her nervousness about tonight. It had been a good day, culminating now, as she readied herself for the evening.

With Gwen's help she had put on her new dress. It felt and fit superbly. The black silk dress was elegant, baring one shoulder and covering the other in a sweeping arc of silk that crisscrossed and supported her breasts, lifting them to show their fullness yet not making her seem overly bold. The dress accented her slim waist before it flared over her hips, ending in a slightly ruffled hem that was more an irregular arc than a closed circle. It had a split side that gave brief glimpses of calf and thigh with each step she took.

Heather hoped she looked as good in the dress as Gwen had said she did. She knew she felt good wearing it, although at the same time she hoped she wasn't being too conspicuous. She admitted she was not used to wearing such a daring dress, but she had once again deferred to Gwen. After all, she reasoned, it was a special night and she wanted to look the part.

To finish off the look, a single string of pearls surrounded her neck and a cluster of three pearls on golden chains hung enticingly from each ear. The jewelry was Gwen's. Her friend insisted she wear the pearls tonight.

Eschewing formal makeup, Heather applied a deeper blue eye shadow than she normally used, this time at Laureen's insistence. "It will bring out your natural skin tones better under the artificial light in the gallery," which was something Heather readily admitted knowing nothing about. Her shoes were simple black pumps with three-inch heels that she hoped would not make her feet ache too badly before the evening was over.

Snapping her makeup case closed, Heather took a deep breath and stood. She was as ready as she could be to face the first night of her new life.

Halfway to the door, she heard a low knock. "Come in," she called as she stopped walking. The door opened slowly. Heather waited but no one came in, although she could sense eyes staring at her. A strange chill ran the length of her body. "Yes?"

"You look real p-p-pretty, Miss Heather," Gregg Farley said softly.

"Gregg!" A warm, wonderful rush of love surged

through Heather. She walked toward the boy's voice and heard him move toward her. Just as she was reaching out to embrace him, she felt his hand take hers and shake it firmly. Heather paused, flustered for a moment before she remembered Tom telling her weeks ago that Gregg was reaching that funny age of being embarrassed by demonstrations of affection.

"Did you have a nice trip?" she asked, recovering quickly and not holding his hand for too long.

"Did he ever!" declared Emma Kline.

"Emma, you too?" Heather asked, surprised but glad.

"You really didn't think I'd miss this, did you?" Emma asked jovially. "No, of course you didn't," she answered for Heather as she swept the younger woman into her arms.

"Where's Tom?" Heather asked after she hugged Emma and had been released.

"Aw . . . he's still kissin' Gwen," Gregg told her in a strangely subdued voice.

"No he's not," Tom said as he stepped into the now crowded office. "Evenin', Heather," he said as he, too, took her hand. The gentle pressure he exerted made Heather feel good.

"It is a good evening now," she told them, knowing that her eyes were filling with moisture. "Do you like the dress?" she asked as she whirled around, making the ruffled silk fly upward and giving them all a glance of her well-shaped legs while she fought to control her emotions.

"I'll say one thing about it," Emma began, and Heather heard the familiar bantering tones in her friend's voice. "You sure could make a nice living in Tahoe . . ."

"Emma!"

"Only kidding. It's absolutely gorgeous."

"Thank you," Heather said with a slight curtsy.

"Enough compliments," came Gwen's authoritative voice. "We've a party starting in"—she paused to glance at her watch—"exactly eleven minutes, and I don't want her ego any bigger than it is! Shall we go out front?" Gwen asked over the laughs her comment caused.

With Emma's arm linked in hers, Heather followed Gwen and Tom. Inside the large gallery room, Heather called Gregg over to her.

"I know this isn't a rodeo, but would you tell me what everything looks like?"

"Yes, ma'am," he said in a serious voice, knowing with the instinctiveness of an eight-year-old that he was doing something important. As Gregg took a deep breath, Emma's hand covered Heather's and pressed it comfortingly.

"It's kinda a big room, with long white walls." Gregg started slowly, sounding a little self-conscious, but pushed on anyway. "The walls are real shiny, and the floor's wood. I'm not sure what kind . . ."

"Oak," Gwen told him.

"The ceilin's white, too, with lots a small lights comin' out."

"Spotlights," Gwen added.

"And the lights are shinin' on your sclup . . . sculptures. Makes them look real fine. Oh! Wow!" Gregg yelled as his eyes fell on a special display of three bronze busts, one elevated above the other two. "You put me and Dad and Reid together," he said excitedly.

Heather bit down on her lower lip as she fought off the invasion of hurt that just the mention of Reid's name had hit her with. She fought her battle and won as she pushed aside the feeling of betrayal.

"Polaris looks real good," Gregg continued, oblivious to Heather's reaction of seconds ago. At the mention of his name, Polaris barked once, eliciting laughs from everyone. "I'm glad he's the first sculpture you see when you come in. Next to him are those funny-shaped things from the studio walk."

"Abstracts," Gwen informed him at the same time as Heather.

"They're still funny-lookin'," Gregg declared, adamantly refusing to change his mind.

"Thank you, Gregg," Heather said as she pulled her hand from Emma's and began to walk toward one of the abstracts.

"Time," Gwen called as the front door opened and voices began to float to Heather's ears. The next thing she knew, Laureen, Gwen's assistant, was pressing a glass into her hand.

"I don't think I should drink," Heather told her.

"It's not to drink—it's to occupy your hands. That way you'll have something to do with them," she told Heather in a friendly and conspiratorial voice.

Suddenly voices swirled around her, and for a moment Heather's eternal darkness frightened her. There were too many people around her all at once, talking, jabbering, and fighting to give her compliments.

She fought off the fear, smiling all the while as Gwen returned to her side and began to introduce her to the different visitors. By the fifth introduction Heather knew it was pointless to try to remember the names. She just smiled and nodded. The muted strains of bits and pieces of conversations bounced in her ears and several times she smiled at the astonished reactions of those who learned she was blind.

The minutes turned into hours, and as the evening

changed to night, it all became a blur of time in Heather's mind. Halfway through the party, Heather became aware of a new sensation. It was as if she were no longer standing on the gallery floor amidst the people but was a separate entity hovering over the room, hearing everything but being invisible. She drifted among the people, always guided by either Gwen or Laureen, and never once released the now warm glass of white wine.

"Miss Strand," called a man whose voice she did not recognize but which pulled her back into the reality of the gallery.

"Yes?"

"My name is Malcolm Samuels. I have a gallery in New York, and I just wanted you to know that I think you have a great future ahead of you."

"Thank you," Heather said, flushing slightly at the compliment.

"Don't thank me—I make my living judging the talents of artists. I'm just telling you the truth." The art dealer paused for a moment and Heather heard him take a breath. "Would you consider doing commissions?" he asked.

"I don't really know," Heather replied hesitantly.

"I'm not trying to push you or anything, but I've seen the busts you've done and they are truly magnificent. The young boy looks so . . . alive. And the man with the mustache—the feeling you put into his face, the care and detail—the look you captured is marvelous."

"I . . . thank you again," Heather said, reeling from the impact of the man's description of Reid.

"I just wanted you to know I appreciate your work. And I also would like to invite you to have a showing in New York at my gallery," the man stated suddenly, again catching Heather off guard. Laureen's hand tightened in warning on Heather's arm and Heather smiled at the man.

"That would be very nice, but of course it would be up to Gwen," she stated matter-of-factly. "She is my representative."

"Of course," Malcolm Samuels said politely. "I just wanted to know if you'd be interested."

Heather smiled at him but did not miss the slight change in his voice as he had spoken. Although she and Gwen had not yet spoken about a representation contract, Heather had already made up her mind. No matter what Heather's personal problems, she trusted Gwen implicitly.

"Are they all like that?" Heather asked Laureen after Samuels had gone.

"Actually, he's one of the better ones."

"Oh," Heather sighed, wondering again about the world she was entering.

"How're you doing?" Tom Farley asked as his hand replaced Laureen's and guided her away from the main crowd.

"Fine, I guess—a little strange, but I'm doing all right."

"I feel pretty strange myself. I'm not used to these artsy-type people," he admitted.

"They're not that different from the people you worked with before you came to the ranch," Heather said.

"They're different enough," Tom replied, and Heather heard the hidden plea in his voice.

"They're just people, Tom—not any stranger than we. They talk about different things and dress a little fancier, I imagine, but they're just people."

"They are very different than we are, Heather—very much so." Suddenly she knew what was bothering Tom. She stopped for a moment and listened for voices around them. When she felt they were as alone as possible in this crowd, she spoke softly and earnestly to him.

"Tom, you can't let something like this interfere with your feelings. It doesn't matter about these people, the way they talk or dress. The only thing that really matters is the way you feel, the way Gwen feels, and, after that, the way Gregg feels."

Tom did not respond immediately and Heather hoped she hadn't overstepped her boundaries with him. A few seconds later Tom shifted uneasily on his feet and spoke.

"I left this type of life five years ago and I found something that I had been missing. I love working on the ranch and I don't know if I want to leave it."

"No one is asking or telling you to leave it. But you also have to think about the future—yours and Gregg's—and if you want Gwen to be a part of it."

"It's not easy," Tom admitted.

"No, nothing important is. But if you want something badly enough, you have to work hard to make it happen. Part of that work is understanding the other person and the other person's needs."

"Heather, about Reid," Tom began. Heather's breath caught at Tom's mention of his name, but she quickly hid her reaction. "I'm sorry," he said in a low voice. "But I'll remember what you just said, and I'll think on it."

"Please do just that," Heather said, but her mind was still churning from the mention of Reid's name.

Tom started to guide Heather back to the main

crowd, but she stopped for a moment as her fingers brushed against bronze. She realized suddenly that they had been standing next to the pedestal that held the sculptures of Gregg, Tom, and Reid.

Unable to stop herself, her fingers traced over Reid's face for a moment. Far away, she heard Tom call her name. She nodded slowly as she pulled her hand from the bronze and again gripped the glass.

Slowly, as Tom walked with her into the main flow of the party, Heather answered the myriad questions directed at her, smiled, and nodded knowingly at those who talked about well-known artists and their works. Soon she had again reached that wonderful state of separation from those around her as she mingled with the crowd but allowed her mind to float above it all, still fighting deep within her heart to keep the recurring thoughts of Reid Hunter away from her mind.

"Holding up okay?" Gwen whispered into her ear as the party began to dwindle.

"I feel like I'm ten feet tall and growing," Heather replied in a matching whisper. "I find it difficult to believe so many people like my works."

"Why? I already told you they would. And I know! Besides, I have five deposit checks in the office already."

"Five . . ." Heather repeated as she sucked in her breath. "That's good, I think," she said as a feeling of elation rode alongside one of loss for those pieces she would never touch again.

"Good? Good? No, it's not good—it's wonderful!" Gwen stated excitedly. "Heather, it's an excellent start."

"Which ones?"

"*The Unicorn* and four abstracts: *Mother Lode, Desert's Cry, Guinevere,* and *Destiny's Hand,*" Gwen told her.

Heather smiled at first. She had sculpted *The Unicorn* after reading a short story about a magical unicorn and a leprechaun. The work had been fun and the finished product had drawn praise from everyone who had seen it. It stood twenty-seven inches tall and three and a half feet long. Its single horn had tapered almost to the thinness of a small nail. She was glad someone had bought that piece.

The sale of the abstracts surprised her. Usually it took a while before a sculptor was able to sell his abstracts. Abstract collectors wanted the work of artists who already had a good reputation.

"Well?" Gwen prompted after a few minutes.

"I was just wondering why the abstracts sold instead of the realistic pieces."

"Because, my dear innocent, the people can see your talent is not the average. You will become important in the art world, and they want to be in on the ground floor. Abstract sculpture to them is an investment in the future."

"Meaning they buy cheap and sell high." Heather laughed at her words, not really sure if she meant them.

"If you call an average of ten thousand dollars cheap, then yes."

"Ten thousand?" Heather asked, her jaw dropping at Gwen's words.

"Each."

"Don't joke."

"When we discussed pricing, you told me you didn't know a thing about it. You said I should take care of that. I did. *The Unicorn* went for seventy-five hundred.

The abstracts from nine thousand to twelve thousand," Gwen informed Heather in a lilting, superior, yet jocular manner.

"Oh. . . ."

"The five pieces," Gwen continued proudly, "together brought a gross of forty-nine thousand, eight hundred and fifty dollars," she said, lowering her voice so only Heather would hear.

"I . . ." Heather said, trying to adjust to the fact that people would pay that much money for what had given her so much enjoyment.

"That's a good response. Keep it that way in the future," Gwen said as she placed her arm around Heather's waist. "Now, do you believe me?"

"Believe you about what?"

"That you are talented."

"I guess so. . . . This wasn't a fluke?" Heather asked. "It's supposed to take years and years to sell your work for so much."

"That's what I've been trying to tell you. These people who bought tonight, and will buy during the next weeks, are getting a bargain and they know it. Right now your work is selling inexpensively. In a year the price will be . . . I won't even try to guess," Gwen finished, pulling Heather close before releasing her.

As Heather thought about what Gwen had said, the gallery seemed to quiet down magically, and suddenly Heather knew her first show had ended for the night. She felt a wave of calm repose wash over her and breathed a sigh of release. It was over and she had survived. In fact, she had even enjoyed some parts of it.

"Gather 'round everybody," Gwen called. Heather felt Emma's hand on her arm and let her friend guide her. "The party is over and it's time to drink to our success. Where's Gregg?" she asked suddenly, concern edging her voice.

Tom chuckled. "He and Polaris are sound asleep in the corner across from your office."

"Why didn't you put him on the couch in the office?" Gwen asked with motherly concern.

"He was comfortable and out of the way, and he wanted to watch everything. He's fine," Tom finished, and Heather heard the warmth in his voice. She knew it was not just for Gregg either.

"In that case, shall we go on with the celebration?"

Laureen gave everyone glasses and Heather heard a cork pop and they all cheered. Polaris woke, barked several times, and everyone laughed at his joining in. But Heather thought it strange that he didn't come over to them. *Too many strangers,* she thought.

After the champagne was poured, they held their glasses high, each person touching Heather's glass first and then each other's.

"To the continued success and long career of Miss Heather Strand, *artiste extraordinaire!*" Gwen toasted.

"Amen," came Tom's reply, quickly followed by everyone elses.

Heather took a long sip from her glass, enjoying the feel of bubbles bursting at her nose and liking the chilled dry taste of the champagne. Suddenly she felt tired and, one at a time, she kicked off the black pumps. No sooner had she finished her first glass than she felt it being refilled.

"No more," she pleaded. "I'm getting dizzy already."

"Get used to it," Gwen ordered. "This is only the beginning. And in the future try to eat something during the day!"

"I think I have a lot to get used to," Heather

responded, and smiled, but took only the barest sip of champagne. She felt a wave of sadness and tried to shake it away. "I think I'd like to change into my regular clothing now. I'm feeling really bushed," she said as she turned and began walking to the office.

As Heather opened the office door, she heard the front door open and close. Suddenly Polaris barked.

"Polaris," she called. The large shepherd was between her and the front door, but did not come immediately to her. The people behind her saw the dog hesitate, its tail wagging. "Polaris!" she called again. Polaris finally turned and came to Heather's side.

"It took you long enough," she said in a low, chiding voice. "Heel," she ordered as she stepped into the office. Shrugging, Heather closed the office door, and before undressing she sat on the couch and breathed a sigh of relief. She hadn't realized how tired her feet and legs were. The opening-night party was not an easy task, but it was thrilling just the same, she thought. There had been only one thing missing, but *he* would be missing forever.

Gwen watched Heather's retreating back until she heard the door open. Then Laureen tugged on her elbow. She looked, and froze, as did everyone else. Her eyes widened momentarily as the man stepped into the light. Hazel eyes met hazel eyes and suddenly everyone in the gallery stopped breathing. Gwen saw Reid look at her and then at the others. He stayed silent as he watched Heather close the door to the office.

Slowly, purposefully, Reid nodded to everyone and began to walk to the door that Heather had disappeared behind. As he crossed the small space, Reid was conscious of the looks of disbelief on everyone's faces, but he no longer cared what anyone thought or said. He had only one thing on his mind. Nothing else mattered.

"Here we go," muttered Emma in a low voice as Reid opened the office door and stepped inside.

Chapter Twenty-two

Sighing gently, as if the sigh could give her strength, Heather decided she must make her tired body move. It was time to change out of the dress and to leave the gallery for the night. Before she could gather enough energy to stand, she heard the office door open and close. Polaris stayed at her feet, but she felt his tail wag. She waited to hear a voice, but there was only silence.

"Yes?" she asked, expecting either Emma or Gwen to reply.

"You look lovely tonight, but that doesn't compensate for your lack of manners. Hasn't anyone ever told you it's impolite to hang up in the middle of a conversation?" Heather felt a rush of dizziness sweep through her at the sound of Reid's voice, but her fast-rising anger pushed the feeling aside.

"I was finished with the conversation. I said what was necessary. Now, get out of here!" she ordered as she stood and faced the direction his voice came from.

"I wasn't finished," he told her in a low voice, "and I'm going to have my say."

"I told you I didn't want to speak with you again. I want you out of my life. I mean it! Reid, leave me alone!" she cried desperately, trying to control her emotions and to still the voice in her heart that called her words lies.

"No."

"Damn you, Reid," she said in a voice that cracked with anger. She heard him step toward her and she backed away. *No*, her mind screamed, *stay away from me. Don't touch me. . . .* But she couldn't voice these cries; her tongue was paralyzed. She heard him come closer; she could feel the heat of his body as he neared her. "No. . . . Reid. . . ." His hand, burning hot, touched her shoulder.

"I love you," he said, his mouth hovering near hers.

Heather shook his hand from her skin, angry at her inability to rid herself of this destructive desire for him that had returned with his touch.

"You don't love me. If you did, there would have been no lies," she said in a whisper.

"I didn't have any choice. I tried to stop what was happening to us. I tried, but I couldn't," he told her honestly.

"So you made me become part of your lie? You made me live the lie for five months?" she spat, acid flowing in her words. The hurt and pain she had been attempting to bottle up broke forth, boiling upward, freed by his declaration of love.

"I was wrong," Reid stated with no attempt to deny her words. He watched her face as he spoke and the taut lines that held her lovely features captive. He saw the lines waver as he spoke and watched her blue eyes fill with tears. His heart twisted painfully as his hands balled into ineffective fists of frustration.

"Why?" she asked in a voice so low he almost missed the word.

"We need to talk, to go someplace more private so I can explain everything to you."

Heather knew she was crying. Suddenly Reid's fingers were on her cheeks, wiping away the moisture. Pulling away as if she'd been burned, Heather's back came against the office wall.

"No!" she cried to both Reid and herself. She knew she wanted nothing more than to be with him; she wanted and needed the strength of his arms around her, his lips on hers, but she could not. She would not allow herself to be used and hurt again.

"Tell me you love me," Reid demanded in harsh, clipped words. "Tell me!" Heather tried to deny it, tried to summon the words. But again she could not.

"We still have a chance," Reid said. "Heather, we can make things right."

"Please leave, Reid. I don't want to be hurt anymore," Heather said, turning her tear-streaked face from him. She did not want him looking at her now, while she was unable to hide her tears. She could already imagine the pity that was on his features, and she could not touch his face to know if her fear was real. She stiffened as his fingers cupped her chin and turned her face back to his. Her breath was trapped somewhere between her chest and throat, and her heart hammered wildly.

Reid gazed at Heather as he turned her face to his. Her soft sweet lips were drawn in a tight line, their corners dipping slightly. Her eyes were squeezed shut, but tears continued to flow in uneven paths. Slowly,

Reid leaned forward and kissed her. Then he stepped back and took her hands in his, raising them to his face.

"Look at me—look at me and tell me you don't love me," he ordered.

Forcing her trembling hands to stop by the sheer strength of her will, Heather "looked" at Reid. Her fingertips traced the reality of the features she had been dreaming of since she had left her home. The weathered but unwrinkled skin, the finely chiseled lines of his chin, and the fullness of the lips beneath the soft tickling of his thick mustache were all visible to her fingers. Gazing at him, Heather knew she could no longer deny her love—not while she touched him.

"I love you, Reid," she whispered.

"I know," he said softly.

"But that fact doesn't change anything. I won't live a life of lies. I won't be deceived or deceive anyone. I'm sorry, Reid, but we have no future." Heather spoke, ignoring the sadness and loss that filled her voice, trying to disregard her tears and, above all, the way her heart cried.

"Have you tried to see it from my side?" Reid prodded as he stepped away from her. "Have you thought about how I feel?" he asked in a low voice that did not mask the hardness that warned Heather of his anger.

"I tried. I tried to understand why you did it, but I couldn't."

"No? Perhaps you should have tried harder. I have a question for you." Heather heard him pause, as if he were waiting for her. She nodded her head slowly, chewing her lower lip as she waited. "Would you have hired me if I had come to you as Reid Hunter, one of the owners of the Broadlands Ranch, instead of an unemployed foreman? Would you have considered me if I had told the truth on my resume?"

Heather listened intently to his words, with her heart still pounding and her hands clasped firmly together. He was right, she suddenly realized. She would not have spoken to him at all if he'd put down the truth. No owner of a ranch would want another ranch owner's hands on their property.

"And," Reid continued, "because I lied to you I was able to do the Strand Ranch, you, and even myself a lot of good. That is the truth, isn't it?"

"Yes," Heather answered.

"Since we agree on that, I think you owe me one favor."

"Owe you?" Heather echoed his words in surprise.

"Come with me. Let's talk—let's try to work this out."

Heather felt herself being pulled in opposite directions. She wanted no further pain and hurt, and to do what Reid wanted meant just that. She also wanted to be with him, to believe him and love him. She was afraid of being alone with him, afraid she would give in to whatever he wanted. She was frightened of the return of a pain worse than what she was already living with. She wanted to be safe and secure and not have to worry about what would happen tomorrow.

"I can't," she said at last. "I need some time to think. So much has happened. . . ." She also knew she needed to be strong to avoid more hurt.

"Damn it, Heather! Why won't you listen to reason?" Reid growled.

Again Heather felt his hands on her shoulders pulling her roughly against him. His mouth was on hers and his hands pressed, iron hot, into her soft skin. She felt his lean, hard chest against her own, forcing an onrushing tide of desire to flow over her.

Her breath fled when his mouth reached hers. Memories of their nights of lovemaking poured through her mind, weakening her resolve. She tasted the sweetness of his lips until her world exploded inside her head.

Fighting for her life, Heather drew away from him.

"No more," she pleaded as she tried to control her raging emotions.

"You love me. It's that simple. Now you're coming with me," Reid told her in a steel-tinged voice. His hand on her wrist was an unyielding band.

"No!"

"Yes!" Slowly, Heather felt herself pulled along. When they crossed the office, Heather knew they were going to Gwen's private entrance, not to the door that led to the gallery itself. Heather tried to twist free of Reid's grip, but it was too powerful to fight. As she did, she heard Polaris's low growl of warning, which turned into a confused whine at the sight of her and Reid.

"Sit!" Reid commanded the dog. "Stay." Heather heard another low whine of protest but did not hear Polaris move. Then the doorlatch clicked open and she felt the cool night air rush across her face and shoulders.

"Please, Reid, let me go," she pleaded. "My shoes!" she cried as she stepped on a small pebble.

"Not until we've talked. Afterward you can do whatever you want," he told her as he lifted her and carried her bodily across the parking lot.

Heather leaned against the leather headrest, trying to sort out the thoughts that paraded through her mind. It had been at least twenty minutes since they'd driven from the parking lot—twenty minutes of listening to the wind rush past the windshield.

She was drained, emotionally and physically. She was too tired to fight anymore; she just wanted this ordeal over with. Yet, at the same time, she wondered what Reid had in mind. She thought she knew him well. She was not afraid physically—perhaps that was why she had not called out for help.

"Where are we going?"

"Someplace where we won't be disturbed."

"So you can take full advantage of me?" she asked, her voice laced with a sarcasm she hadn't meant.

"If that's what you want to think," Reid said tersely.

"Talk to me now," she asked.

"No. I want to look at you, I want to hold your hand, and afterward I . . ." Reid stopped short of saying what was on his mind, but the way Heather shifted in the seat told him she had understood.

Heather could not respond to the last statement. She knew what he meant. Yes, she wanted to make love to Reid for the rest of her life, but his actions had put a stop to that possibility. *Why couldn't he have been more honest with me?* Why hadn't he said anything after they had become lovers? His pride, Gwen had said. Damn his stupid masculine pride!

"How much longer?"

"Half hour," Reid said as he glanced quickly at her and then back to the road. The speedometer needle was resting on the ninety mark and had been since they'd left Santa Fe. The highway was deserted and Reid wanted to get to his destination as soon as possible. His confident hands held the Mercedes' wheel in a sure grip. His driving wasn't reckless; whenever he saw headlights approaching, he slowed until the car was passed.

Reid was tired; it had been a long day and he knew it would be an even longer night. But when it was over he hoped he would be proved right in what he'd done.

"Reid?" Heather asked in a faraway voice.

"Yes?"

"What kind of car is this?" Reid smiled at the question.

"A Mercedes. Why?"

"I've never ridden in a car like this. It's so quiet and feels so solid. I didn't know you could rent this type."

"You can't around here."

"Oh. . . ." Heather waited but Reid did not elaborate. The smooth ride and the constant hum of the wind had a calming effect on Heather's mind. Without realizing it, she fell asleep.

Nearing their destination, Reid slowed the car and glanced at Heather. He had been aware of the change in her breathing and had known she'd fallen into a light sleep.

Reid slowed the car further and turned off the main highway fifteen miles outside of Albuquerque. He knew this road like the back of his hand and could not stop the smile that spread across his face as he drove. Five minutes later he pulled the silver car to a halt in front of a small cabin.

Reid leaned across the seats and gently turned Heather's face to his. He kissed her lips lightly and drew away.

The changing rhythm of the car and the distinct difference of the new road's surface had awakened Heather, but she did not let Reid know it. She kept her breathing at a steady pace and even when the car stopped did not betray herself. Reid's fingers on her chin startled her, but his lips were soft and gentle. Slowly, she let her breathing return to normal.

"We're here," Reid said.

"Wherever here is." Silently, Reid got out of the car. Heather's door opened and she took his hand as she, too, stood. Beneath her feet was the velvet softness of sodded grass. Heather was very conscious of Reid's hand on her elbow and the heat that spread from his touch. The occasional meeting of their hips as he guided her added a strange, almost ethereal quality to the night. Reid stopped for a moment and the sound of a lock being opened reverberated in the still night air.

Stepping inside, Heather became immediately aware of the dormant quality of the air. *Not dormant but unused,* she thought as her finely tuned senses filtered everything. This place had been aired out recently, but the older heaviness had not yet gone.

"Are you going to tell me where we are?" she asked with a hint of impatience in her voice. It had been a long day and a long night. She had been up and down enough times in one day to fray the staunchest of nervous systems, and Heather readily admitted she was not in that class.

"Heather," Reid said as he took her hand in his. "First, understand that I love you."

Heather nodded her head slowly, again trying to fight this new assault to the emotion brought on by his words. His hand pressed hers tightly.

"Would you like a drink?"

"No!" Heather yelled loudly. "What I want is for you to stop torturing me. Tell me what you have to say. But stop this insanity. Where are we?"

"Sit," he said.

"My name is Heather, not Polaris!"

"On the couch, not the floor," he retorted.

"Reid . . ." she said ineffectually as she gave up and sat.

"We're at Broadlands." Heather's breath caught as she heard the words. Her mind again became jumbled. Why had he brought her to his ranch? No, not his ranch anymore, she thought sadly. Heather heard Reid begin to pace in front of her as she sat back. She knew he was getting ready to speak, and she had every intention of listening. She needed to hear his words now, almost as much as she needed to touch him and feel the fire that he could create within her.

"You know most of the story already. When I got out of the service, I came home a different man than the one who had left. I needed some time to adjust and to understand what had happened to me and my ideals.

"But when I got home and tried to tell Patrick about my experiences, he turned a deaf ear to me. He told me I had made a decision, one he had not agreed with, and now I had to live with it. In the meantime, he expected me to forget the war and get back to working on the ranch.

"I tried, but it was no good. Every morning I woke from the same nightmare. Every night I went to sleep knowing what waited for me. It was no good trying to talk to Pat. All he was interested in was the ranch.

"I had lost all my feelings for the ranch and decided to try to find myself. I signed over my part of the ranch to Pat with the understanding that if and when I had come to terms with myself I would return. But I knew that would never be. I no longer wanted the easy things, the things that had been given to me. I felt I didn't deserve them and I think Pat felt the same way. He wouldn't talk to me for four years, and when he finally did, it was because of Gwen, and we had another bad fight that caused an even deeper division between us."

Reid paused for a moment and Heather had a chance

to think. The words he was speaking seemed to tunnel into her mind and build a platform for her to start to understand him. She knew that what he was doing was not easy; that much she was able to tell from his voice.

"I founded the New Life Foundation with Mike Bloom. I gave them the trust fund that my father had left me. It was enough to start the Foundation and it helped me to think I was making up for some of the pain I had caused.

"I gave the Foundation every penny I had and then started out as a plain cowboy with no background other than what I had invented. It was an easy life—there were no problems, no headaches, and no responsibilities to anyone other than myself and the ranch owner I was working for."

"But that wasn't enough," Heather stated.

"No, it wasn't. I learned I liked responsibility, but not the kind that was always forced on me, like the ranch, and the men who were in my platoon. I enjoyed the responsibilities I earned by working for them. I built myself from cowboy to foreman, and I was happy. Then I met you."

Heather heard the words and a chill ran along her spine. She held her breath, waiting for him to continue and trying to push aside the pain she felt for him with each admission he made.

"The moment I saw you, I knew I should have turned and run. I couldn't. You were too beautiful. I took the job, but I tried to avoid you. It was plain to see that the ranch needed guidance and I threw myself into it. But every day I saw you, and every day I fell more and more in love. It was then that I began to regret what I had cast aside ten years ago."

"But if you hadn't, you would not have met me."

"Yes I would. I don't know how, but I think we were

destined to meet and fall in love." Heather refused to let the tears his words called up escape. She must listen carefully and be rational. Too much was at stake for her.

"My biggest mistake was not being honest with you, in letting you find out the truth before I could tell you."

"Why did you wait?"

"Because once the lies started, they kept building up. I was going to tell you the truth, and I was going to ask you to marry me just before Gwen came to the ranch. Up to that point, I was still a ranch owner, even if I had turned my back on it.

"But Gwen had come to tell me that Patrick was in deep trouble. Gwen and I decided that we owed my father our loyalty even if we didn't agree with Patrick. When I came back to the ranch after seeing Patrick, I was truly what I had told you I was. I no longer owned anything. I was just a foreman."

Heather let out a deep breath and stood. She had listened to Reid and absorbed everything. Now she was mad.

"So you couldn't trust your emotions, could you? You couldn't come to me and tell me what had happened. You had to stand on your arrogant male pride and be the brave man who turned away the love he was offered. Just who the hell do you think you are, Reid Hunter?"

"Just a man," he said.

"No, you're not *just* a man. You're my man!" Heather stated before she could control her tongue. She stopped then, her hand covering her mouth as if she were trying to put the words back.

"I didn't want people to talk about you, to say I married you for your ranch."

"I don't give a damn what anyone has to say. I never

did and I never will. I fell in love with Reid Hunter, not what Reid Hunter does for a living, not what the size of Reid Hunter's portfolio is, nor what Reid Hunter's past was. I fell in love with you because you are you. Can't you understand that?'' she asked in a hoarse whisper.

"I did, twice. The first time was when I understood what you had said to me. I know what the one thing is that I have that's most important to you, that's more important than my being your social equal. And I realized it again last night when you hung up on me and I found myself losing you."

"You did?"

"Yes. My love and need for you! When you hung up on me, I told Tom I was leaving for a few days and he was to assign whoever he damn well wanted to take charge of the ranch. Then I went to Tahoe and chartered a private plane. I landed in Albuquerque this morning."

Sitting was the only thing that Heather could do. She didn't trust her legs to support her as she heard Reid's revelations.

"After listening to what you had to say, I knew that if I wanted you I had to do more than just come after you. I had too many things still hanging over my head.

"When I landed in Albuquerque, I came here, to Broadlands. I met with Pat, and we spent the morning yelling and screaming at each other. When it was over, I apologized to him—not for leaving in the first place, but for not being able to tell him why."

"That must have been hard," Heather said, knowing the strength of Reid's will and imagining that of his twin brother's.

"Yes it was, but it was necessary. He's my brother, and I wanted a brother again." Heather felt the sting of tears in her eyes, but this time did not fight them.

"Pat and I built this cabin," Reid said in a soft voice. "We built this one for me and another for Pat over the first two summer breaks from college. These cabins were our own, the first things we'd ever done without our father's help. We used the money we earned working as cowhands on the ranch.

"Pat and I talked about all of this today. Just before I left for Santa Fe, Pat asked me to come back."

Heather waited again, knowing intuitively what Reid had told Pat.

"I thanked him. Then I told him I have a new home, if everything works out. Then I drove to Santa Fe."

"I'm glad," Heather said.

"That I came to Santa Fe?"

"That you came home and found you had a brother again."

"Heather," Reid began. Heather heard the change in his voice and felt her body react to it. "Will you marry me?"

"You're not afraid of what people will say?" she asked, half in jest, half in truth.

"I only care what you have to say."

"No more pride? No more cowboy creed? No, don't answer that. I don't think you would be Reid Hunter without those things," Heather said. She knew she was talking a lot to cover the sudden nervousness that had overtaken her. She needed to talk in order to think.

Then she could no longer talk or think as Reid pulled her to her feet and kissed her. Her arms went around him and pressed him tightly to her. The kiss lasted an eternity, until Heather could not think but only feel.

She felt Reid lift her and carry her across the room and up several steps. His lips stayed glued to hers as he moved. She felt the softness of a feather mattress beneath her when Reid finally loosened his grip.

"This dress should be declared illegal," he murmured in her ear as his hand slipped under the silk and cupped her breast. Fire, heat, and desire ebbed and flowed through her as his hands renewed their aquaintance with her body.

Heather smiled as Reid's lips went to her neck and her fingers wound through his hair. This is where she wanted to be—this is where she belonged.

Reid undressed her quickly, and when he finally joined her on the bed, his body was as bare as hers. Heather kissed him deeply, tasting his lips and then moving her tongue along the side of his neck. It was as if she could not get enough of his taste and she knew she never would. She would spend a lifetime trying.

Suddenly Reid was poised above her, his mouth inches from her ear, the heat from his body searing hers along its length. Her hands were on his back, urging him to her, but he held back.

"Answer me!" he said in a low, steel-tinged voice.

"I thought I had," she told him as her hands stroked his back.

"Say it!"

"Yes! Yes! Yes!" she cried. Only then did they join and become one.

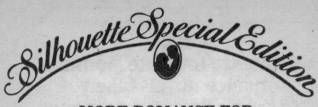

MORE ROMANCE FOR
A SPECIAL WAY TO RELAX
$1.95 each

2 ☐ Hastings	21 ☐ Hastings	41 ☐ Halston	60 ☐ Thorne
3 ☐ Dixon	22 ☐ Howard	42 ☐ Drummond	61 ☐ Beckman
4 ☐ Vitek	23 ☐ Charles	43 ☐ Shaw	62 ☐ Bright
5 ☐ Converse	24 ☐ Dixon	44 ☐ Eden	63 ☐ Wallace
6 ☐ Douglass	25 ☐ Hardy	45 ☐ Charles	64 ☐ Converse
7 ☐ Stanford	26 ☐ Scott	46 ☐ Howard	65 ☐ Cates
8 ☐ Halston	27 ☐ Wisdom	47 ☐ Stephens	66 ☐ Mikels
9 ☐ Baxter	28 ☐ Ripy	48 ☐ Ferrell	67 ☐ Shaw
10 ☐ Thiels	29 ☐ Bergen	49 ☐ Hastings	68 ☐ Sinclair
11 ☐ Thornton	30 ☐ Stephens	50 ☐ Browning	69 ☐ Dalton
12 ☐ Sinclair	31 ☐ Baxter	51 ☐ Trent	70 ☐ Clare
13 ☐ Beckman	32 ☐ Douglass	52 ☐ Sinclair	71 ☐ Skillern
14 ☐ Keene	33 ☐ Palmer	53 ☐ Thomas	72 ☐ Belmont
15 ☐ James	35 ☐ James	54 ☐ Hohl	73 ☐ Taylor
16 ☐ Carr	36 ☐ Dailey	55 ☐ Stanford	74 ☐ Wisdom
17 ☐ John	37 ☐ Stanford	56 ☐ Wallace	75 ☐ John
18 ☐ Hamilton	38 ☐ John	57 ☐ Thornton	76 ☐ Ripy
19 ☐ Shaw	39 ☐ Milan	58 ☐ Douglass	77 ☐ Bergen
20 ☐ Musgrave	40 ☐ Converse	59 ☐ Roberts	78 ☐ Gladstone

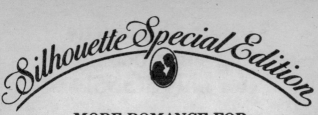

MORE ROMANCE FOR
A SPECIAL WAY TO RELAX

$2.25 each

79 ☐ Hastings	84 ☐ Stephens	89 ☐ Meriwether	94 ☐ Barrie
80 ☐ Douglass	85 ☐ Beckman	90 ☐ Justin	95 ☐ Doyle
81 ☐ Thornton	86 ☐ Halston	91 ☐ Stanford	96 ☐ Baxter
82 ☐ McKenna	87 ☐ Dixon	92 ☐ Hamilton	
83 ☐ Major	88 ☐ Saxon	93 ☐ Lacey	

LOOK FOR _WILD IS THE HEART_ BY ABRA TAYLOR
AVAILABLE IN JULY AND
THUNDER AT DAWN BY PATTI BECKMAN IN
AUGUST.

SILHOUETTE SPECIAL EDITION, Department SE/2
1230 Avenue of the Americas
New York, NY 10020

Please send me the books I have checked above. I am enclosing $_____
(please add 50¢ to cover postage and handling. NYS and NYC residents
please add appropriate sales tax). Send check or money order—no cash or
C.O.D.'s please. Allow six weeks for delivery.

NAME _____

ADDRESS _____

CITY _____ STATE/ZIP _____

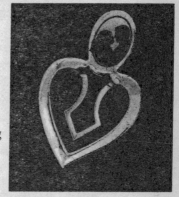

If you enjoyed this book...

...you will enjoy a Special Edition Book Club membership even more.

It will bring you each new title, as soon as it is published every month, delivered right to your door.

15-Day Free Trial Offer

We will send you 6 new Silhouette Special Editions to keep for 15 days absolutely free! If you decide not to keep them, send them back to us, you pay nothing. But if you enjoy them as much as we think you will, keep them and pay the invoice enclosed with your trial shipment. You will then automatically become a member of the Special Edition Book Club and receive 6 more romances every month. There is no minimum number of books to buy and you can cancel at any time.

Get the Silhouette Books Newsletter every month for a year.

Now you can receive the fascinating and informative Silhouette Books Newsletter 12 times a year. Every issue is packed with inside information about your favorite Silhouette authors, upcoming books, and a variety of entertaining features—including the authors' favorite romantic recipes, quizzes on plots and characters, and articles about the locales featured in Silhouette books. Plus contests where you can win terrific prizes.

The Silhouette Books Newsletter has been available only to Silhouette Home Subscribers. Now you, too, can enjoy the Newsletter all year long for just $19.95. Enter your subscription now, so you won't miss a single exciting issue.

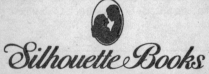